deryck calderwood

Administering and Teaching
Sex Education
in the Elementary School

Muriel Schoenbrun Karlin

Administering and Teaching
Sex Education
in the Elementary School

PARKER PUBLISHING COMPANY, INC.
WEST NYACK, NEW YORK

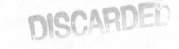

Library of Congress Cataloging in Publication Data

Karlin, Muriel Schoenbrun.
    Administering and teaching sex education in the
elementary school.

    Includes bibliographies.
    1. Sex instruction--United States. 2. Sex
instruction for youth. 3. Sex instruction--Cur-
ricula. I. Title.
HQ57.5.A3K37   372.3'7   75-16480
ISBN 0-13-005165-9

Printed in the United States of America

Lovingly dedicated to
Len, Lisa, Henry and Aline

Why You Need This Book, and How It Will Help You to Establish an Effective Sex Education Program in Your School

The purpose of this book is to provide experienced educators with practical information on tested, existing curricula and programs in sex education. You will find specific guidelines as issued by various states and detailed curricula as furnished by a broad range of school districts. The guidelines, and actual curricula will be invaluable as sources of reliable material you may easily adapt in the formulation of your own plans. This book will help you make certain that your program effectively meets the needs of your students and reflects the wishes of their parents.

There are thousands of sex education programs in schools across the country. They may be called "family living" or even "human sexuality." They may be part of the health education curriculum, the home economics area, social studies, or perhaps taught in an incidental way, namely when children show interest or ask questions. They are varied and dissimilar, due largely to the differences in size or location of the school districts that have developed them.

To obtain the most realistic and best-qualified information, we wrote to the superintendents of education in every one of the fifty states. Many superintendents either sent state-suggested curricula or listed specific programs in various localities. We then contacted each of the respective school districts for further, more detailed information.

A tremendous amount of data resulted, much of which you will find compiled in the pages that follow. However, it is given in the form of practical, tested curricula that you may use or adapt for the primary, intermediate, middle and junior high grades. This will enable you to gear your program more precisely to the wishes of parents, members of the school board, administrators, teachers and yourself.

Statistics, in regard to the efficacy of such programs, e.g., number of pregnancies, rate of venereal disease, before and after, etc., are not available. Many educators who responded also took exception to the request for this type of information because so many factors influence these situations. However, we do know this:

The United States Department of Health, Education and Welfare, in announcing a major program aimed at teaching teenage girls and boys how to become good parents, listed the following:

— Approximately 210,000 girls aged seventeen and under gave birth in the United States last year.
— One of every ten school-age girls is a mother, and sixteen percent of these young mothers have two children.
— The national divorce rate for those married in their teens is three to four times higher than that of any other age group.

However, since sex education is a function of the local community, HEW can only offer recommendations.

In spite of the statistics above, there is still a great deal of controversy in regard to this subject area, with legal prohibitions having been passed in a few states. The Commissioner of Education of one such state wrote: "A few years ago we were faced with open confrontation between those who were for sex education, and those against it in our public schools. After an extended study session by a special committee and after open hearings, our State Board of Education finally decreed that decisions should be made by *local* boards of education as to how they wish to handle such programs of instruction. The State Board did, at that time, offer suggestions and warnings to local boards of education to cover those instances where local school boards decided to include such instruction in their curriculum.

"I think it is fair to say that because of the difficulties that arose regarding sex education, many of our local boards have been steering clear of any involvement. Dependable, practical guidelines are not available. The result is that in many areas, very little is being offered in our public school systems that could be readily identified as sex education, per se. It does, of course, appear in many forms under our comprehensive health education program, biology, homemaking, etc." Thus, the need for this book becomes apparent.

As you read the materials that follow, keep in mind that many localities have borrowed programs, in whole or in part, from other communities, and that their inclusion here is for that same purpose.

The Kingswood Regional High School's statement (Wolfsboro, Vt.) of philosophy is, we feel, very concise, and yet says it all.

It is a basic philosophy of public education to provide each student with an opportunity to develop into a healthy and well-informed adult. Family life education is an essential part of the modern educational curriculum. The school fully realizes the responsibility of the home and church as the primary sources of family life education. The program is designed to *supplement and support* the home and church in family life education. Family life education is a continuous process in which the development of attitudes and understandings are most important. An individual's maturity will contribute toward his self-development and happiness.

In this book, you will find specifics on how to gain acceptance for a sex education program, and practical ways to develop it. You will learn how to set the program in motion, how to choose a staff and train them to teach it. You will be shown how to constantly evaluate the program. A large portion of the book actually describes a *full curriculum*—both concepts *and* actual activities for the primary, middle, intermediate and junior high grades. This is augmented by guidelines that show you how to vary this program to suit the needs of children in *your* school. Since effective communication with parents is vital to the success of any sex education program, there is a full chapter devoted to this subject. As an added practical feature, there is a helpful listing of books, texts, and audio-visual aids that will provide you with supplementary teaching material.

The topics you will cover, the amount of detail, even the approaches you may elect to use will vary, but the goal of giving your children education for a fuller, happier life never changes. This book can help you achieve that goal.

Muriel Schoenbrun Karlin

Acknowledgments

Our sincere thanks to educators from every state of the Union who were kind enough to respond to our requests for information and curricula.

We are especially grateful to the following boards of education: State of Connecticut, State of Delaware, State of Illinois, State of Iowa, State of Kansas, State of Pennsylvania, State of Michigan, Anchorage School District, City of New York, and Parsippany-Troy Hills Township, New Jersey.

Special thanks are due to:
Ms. Nita Rogers, Belleville Public Schools, Belleville, Illinois.
Dr. Ruth V. Byler, Connecticut State Department of Education.
Independent School District #77, Mankato, Minnesota, which provided the curriculum that forms the basis of this book.

One of the joys of preparing this manuscript has been the cooperation of educators across the country who shared information with us. While portions of their material may not be used directly in this volume, their influence was felt most strongly.

On a personal note, grateful thanks are given to Mrs. Jeannette Karlin of Delray Beach, Florida, for typing the manuscript, and to my husband, Dr. Leonard Karlin, for proofreading it and for his constant encouragement.

CONTENTS

Children and youth are constantly asking for help in
facing the many problems related to sexual adjustment
. . . Children and youth want accurate information concerning the normal development toward sexual maturity
. . . How to use statistics (national) to show the need for
a sex education program . . . Teenage marriages . . .
Divorce among teenagers and among individuals who
married during their teens . . . Illegitimate births . . .
Venereal disease . . . Children and youth receive most
sex education from their peers, not their parents . . .
Why concerned parents often feel a strong need for
providing sex education in the school . . . The sex
education program should give your children the specific
information they want and need to know . . . The sex
education program in the schools should provide an
opportunity to reach parents and assist them with their
questions.

Steps in organizing a family life and sex education

Chapter 2 *(continued)*

program . . . Development of initial interest . . . Informal
exploratory committee . . . Community planning committee . . . Determining the specific needs . . . Administrative follow-through . . . Establishing a lay committee
to serve as an advisory group . . . Making a study to
determine the type of program the parents will endorse
. . . How to establish the objectives that will meet the needs
of your students . . . The work of the curriculum committee . . . Establishing the scope of the sex education
program . . . Keeping parents and citizens of the community informed of the entire curriculum.

Determining the role of sex education in the school curriculum . . . Placing the program in the health education
area . . . Placing the program in the subject areas . . .
Sample science and health education unit . . . Selecting
staff for the program . . . Providing strong administrative leadership . . . Special training for teachers , . . .
Continuing inservice education . . . Selecting texts and
audio-visual materials . . . Obtaining community and
parental approval for the program . . . Initiating the
program.

Notifying parents about the particular curriculum being
used . . . The sample letter and curriculum brochure you
may use as a guide . . . Permission forms are a must . . .
Parent workshops in sex education . . . Inviting parental
observation . . . Involving parents in the actual program
. . . Rap sessions with teachers or counselors for parents
who need them . . . Referrals to appropriate agencies.

Levels of psychosexual development . . . The four- to five-year-old . . . The six- to eight-year-old.

Primary Grades—Curriculum Outline

For very young children:

Unit I. Routine Toilet Procedures. Introducing scientific names for parts of the body and bodily functions . . . Helping children to develop acceptable bathroom habits . . . Helping children to develop wholesome attitudes toward the body.

Unit II. The Nature and Purpose of the Family. To bring children into the world and care for them . . . To shape personalities, develop values, habits, and attitudes toward life . . . To provide love, companionship, security, and protection for its members . . . To guide individual members to understand, respect, and accept themselves . . . To provide necessary food, shelter, and physical (material) needs for all its members . . . To provide opportunities for the acceptance of responsibility and learning of respect for others . . . To provide moral and spiritual values.

For young children:

Where Babies Come From. Both mother and father have roles in reproduction . . . Prenatal growth and birth is a miraculous process . . . Human reproduction has deep meaning.

Growth and Development in Boys and Girls. Boys and girls must have a concept of their role in society . . . Each person must discover and develop his self-concept . . . Each person needs to be able to identify and understand the purpose of his external genitalia.

The curriculum

Levels of psychosexual development . . . The nine- to ten-year-old.

Middle Grades—Curriculum Outline

Understanding of and Respect for Reproductive Organs. Each person needs to be able to locate and identify his reproductive organs . . . Each person must understand the danger of injury to his reproductive organs . . . Each person must recognize and take precautionary measures against invasions of his personal privacy by persons other than his parents or medical personnel.

The Need for Families as a Basic Unit of Human Life. The family is a basic unit of human living . . . The family brings children into the world and prepares them for adulthood . . . The family provides moral and spiritual guidance . . . The family furnishes values and ideals . . . The family develops a self-concept within each member . . . The family preserves its heritage . . . The family fosters consideration and sensitivity to feelings of others . . . The family helps the child relate to society and to the world community . . . The family provides sex education.

The curriculum

Levels of psychosexual development . . . The eleven- to thirteen-year-old.

Intermediate Grades—Curriculum Outline

The Anatomy and Physiology of the Human Reproductive System. There are glands that affect your growth . . . All parts of the reproductive system have a definite function . . . There are normal processes of the reproductive system . . . Correct terminology.

Chapter 7 *continued*

Human Reproduction. Male sex cells are produced . . .
The sperm journeys to meet the ovum during mating
. . . Female sex cells are produced . . . The miracle of
life begins when the sperm and ovum meet . . . Prenatal
growth occurs in the uterus . . . Birth occurs . . . Correct
terminology.

The curriculum

Levels of psychosexual development . . . The fourteen- to
sixteen-year-old.

Junior Grades–Curriculum Outline

Unit I. Understanding Adolescent Changes. Stages of
development . . . Body structure . . . Body and mind
relationship . . . Importance of good mental health . . .
Endocrine system . . . Growth spurt . . . Secondary sex
characteristics . . . New feelings and experiences.

The curriculum

Unit II. Young People's Problems in Society. Basic
groups of society . . . Family problems . . . Peer group
behavior . . . Education and its effect on the life of the
individual . . . Dating . . . Religion or philosophy of life
. . . Alcohol, narcotics, and tobacco . . . Premarital
physical sex . . . Venereal diseases.

The curriculum continued

Scope and sequence of the sex education program . . .
Sample lessons . . . Determining other topics to include
. . . Introducing the mental health aspect . . . The prob-
lem of divorce; its effect on the wife and husband and

Chapter 9 *continued*

on young children . . . The role of counseling in the sex
education program.

Establishing guidelines for evaluation of the sex education program . . . Basic steps in evaluation . . . Who
should do the evaluation? . . . Teacher's analysis of sex
education program . . . Pupil evaluations . . . Evaluation
by parents through questionnaires and through comments made casually to teachers, counselors, or administrators . . . Evaluation by administrators . . . Staff
evaluation . . . Surveying the progress of the program
. . . Changes in student attitudes.

Administering and Teaching
Sex Education
in the Elementary School

CHAPTER 1 *How to Gain Acceptance for Launching a Sex Education Program*

There are few programs in the educational milieu today that invite as much diverse opinion as the area of sex education. School officials are being confronted with this topic by parents, clergy, physicians and citizens at large; some demanding, others encouraging; some knowledgeable, others misinformed; some questioning, others criticizing. The many media of communication have served to educate, publicize, condemn and at times misinterpret the role of schools in sex education.

Parents and educators have become acutely aware of the place that sex has assumed in the entertainment media, advertising, fashion, books and magazines. It is a fact that few segments of our society have escaped some sort of involvement with the symbol of sex.

Therefore, it would appear that today's youth are finding themselves enmeshed in emotional and physiological sexual confrontations, not unique necessarily to their generation, but perhaps engaging them in a more open and greater scope than immediate past generations have experienced.

There is an obvious national concern over increasing venereal disease rates, abortion, the new morality, premarital promiscuity, contraception and free love. While these problems need and deserve the careful application of sensitive and mature deliberation, they have all too frequently been the subject of illogical and irrational attacks upon sex education in the schools.

There seems to be little question that sex education is a responsibility that should be shared by the home, church, school and community. Yet it appears clear that the school has a fundamental role to perform. In a concerned effort to assist young people and confront the physiological, psychological, social and ethical implications of sexuality, the schools must assume a definite responsibility for assuring that opportunities prevail through which accurate information and trained leadership are available. Central to such responsibility are opportunities to make mature choices based on facts relative to competing codes of conduct, the implications of one's sex role, planned subject matter in the curriculum that increases in complexity as individual levels of maturity and comprehension increase. Objectives for programs of sex education should be specified by developmental levels. These objectives should be flexible, realistic and coordinated in a manner designed to encourage children to develop a normal progression of interest in and an increasing body of knowledge about human beings and their relationships, with the underlying goal of causing children and youth to form acceptable values and to make wise decisions about their behavior. Sex education can and should be presented from many perspectives; it should grow as the child grows and widen as his experiences widen. There should be no attempt to teach it as an isolated course of study.[1]

Children and Youth Are Asking for Help to Face the Many Problems Related to Sexual Adjustment

In a book entitled *Teach Us What We Want to Know,* Byler, Lewis and Totman report on a survey taken among 5,000 students in Connecticut schools. In the summary, the section "About Sex Education," the authors state:

They [the children] recommended strongly that primary grade children should learn about sex characteristics from raising and studying animals, fish, and other pets. They should have their questions answered in a straightforward and

---

[1] *Guidelines for Sex Education in Public Schools of Pennsylvania.* Reprinted by Parker Publishing Company, Inc., by permission of the Pennsylvania Department of Education.

honest way. In grades 5-6, girls especially need to learn about menstruation in order to allay curiosity and fear, and to prevent embarrassment and other trouble. Boys need to understand about menstruation so they will not ask silly questions.

Sexual relationships should be discussed as early as grade six, says a student. "I know some kids that started then, and there's no stopping them." The major study of sexual development, relations, and behavior should be placed in grades 7 and 8 to prevent experimentation and illegitimacy due to ignorance. "Unless it is taught early," say students, "it won't do any good." It should be accompanied by discussion of the choice of friends, of dating and going steady. Students should be told about the dangers of venereal disease. Pregnancy and birth control should also be taught in grade 7, and again in grade 12 in a course on preparation for marriage. Seniors should learn about genetics and birth, and birth abnormalities and their causes.[2]

In the section about mental health, certainly a related area, the children had this to say:

They think young children should be helped to control their emotions, especially anger and crying; children in grades 3-6 should study how the mind and emotions work; in grades 7-9, as part of understanding the self, students should learn about maturity of behavior and ways of coping with individual problems: "They should learn to face life and its problems."[3]

Earlier marriage and a growing number of teenage divorces present a series of new problems for our young people. The various displays of sex symbols constantly expose them to a variety of stimuli regarding the use and place of sex in life. Because of these many factors in our society, the school needs to assist the home and church in helping youth to be aware of the

[2]Byler, R., G. Lewis and R. Totman, *Teach Us What We Want to Know.* Connecticut State Board of Education. Published by Mental Health Materials Center, Inc., New York, N.Y. Used by permission.

[3]Byler, Lewis, and Totman. *Teach Us What We Want to Know.*

need to develop a responsible personal moral code. The personal counseling that should be part of this program can also help youth face important decisions regarding their sexual behavior. Young people often realize they need such counseling. They must have some place to turn. But even for the young person who is not particularly troubled, information must be made available to him or her to prevent problems from developing.

Children and Youth Want Accurate Information Concerning the Normal Development Toward Sexual Maturity

No two individuals develop physically or mentally at the same rate. Yet comparisons are often made. Boys whose stature is small sometimes become upset when they are twelve or thirteen years old. They find they are smaller than girls of similar age. There is a very valid reason for this. According to statistics, most girls mature in the year between twelve and thirteen. Most boys mature in the year from fourteen to fifteen. Knowledge of this simple fact can alleviate much anxiety. We have heard sighs of relief from the boys, not once but many times. Can you imagine how much anxiety is attached to sexual development and maturation?

The advent of puberty is a time when the adolescent is filled with many feelings and emotions that need explanation. Children should be given information about it long before it occurs. How traumatic it can be for a girl to begin menstruating before she has been taught about it. You might say, "But that should be the parents' responsibility." Certainly, it should. But there are mothers who never teach it—and children without mothers! It should be the school's role to fill any informational gaps. Education is education—be it in reading, arithmetic or in personal matters. We have been bombarded with pleas to make education relevant. What can be more so than wholesome sex education?

Accurate information can help fortify youth against exploitation by others or against the miseries of their bodies. Sex education should lead to more wholesome attitudes. We should, however, insure that such education is accurate and wholesome and that no child is embarrassed or ever made uncomfortable by it.

How to Use Statistics to Show
the Need for a Sex Education Program

Perhaps no greater plea for an effective sex education program can be made than to ask members of your community to look at the statistics in regard to teenage marriage and divorce, illegitimate births and venereal disease. The statistics we are citing below were supplied by the Public Health Service of the Department of Health, Education and Welfare, 5600 Fishers Lane, Rockville, Maryland. These are the latest figures available for the type of information included. They are taken from the publication "Data from the National Vital Statistics System, Vital and Health Statistics" Series 21, Number 23 entitled "Teenagers: Marriages, Divorces, Parenthood, and Mortality," DHEW Publication No. (HRA) 74-1901, and dated August, 1973.

Teenage Marriages

According to the census, there are more teenagers in the United States today than ever before in the history of the country. In 1969 there were an estimated 18.6 million persons fifteen through nineteen years of age. This was nearly 8 million more than in 1949, and 5.6 million more than in 1959. According to the current projections, the teenage population should be in the neighborhood of 25 million by the year 2,000.

Early marriage is more common now than it was at the turn of the century, but slightly less common than it was twenty years ago. About one-third of the women and fourteen percent of the men who married during 1969 were teenagers. An estimated 717,000 women and 311,000 men married at ages under twenty years. This was more than for any of the previous four years and an increase over 1960 of 160,000 women and 110,000 men. The number of teenage marriages was up nearly thirty percent for women and over fifty percent for men in 1969 as compared with 1960. If no significant changes occur in the teenage marriage rate, the number of teenage marriages will continue to increase at a diminishing rate until the late seventies. By then the downward trend in births that began in 1958 and continued through the sixties will have ended this postwar wave of teenage eligibles. (See Tables 1 and 2.)

Table 1. Estimated number and rate of marriages, by age and sex: United States, 1969

[Rates per 1,000 unmarried population in specified group]

	Female		Male	
Age	Number	Rate	Number	Rate
Total ------------	2,145,000	80.0	2,145,000	98.7
15-19 years -----------	717,000	87.7	311,000	34.6
20-24 years -----------	843,000	273.5	985,000	221.1
25-34 years -----------	311,000	189.7	491,000	234.1
35-44 years -----------	129,000	86.0	163,000	123.5
45-54 years -----------	84,000	38.4	101,000	73.2
55-64 years -----------	43,000	14.2	56,000	48.7
65 years and over -------	19,000	2.7	39,000	16.4

Table 2. Median age of spouse, by specified age of teenage bride or groom at first marriage of both: marriage-registration area, 1960-69
[Based on sample data]

Year	Specified age of bride			Specified age of groom		
	Under 18 years	18 years	19 years	Under 18 years	18 years	19 years
	Median age of spouse					
1969	19.7	20.6	21.3	17.3	18.1	18.7
1968	19.7	20.6	21.3	17.3	18.2	18.7
1967	19.8	20.5	21.3	17.5	18.2	18.7
1966	19.7	20.5	21.4	17.3	18.2	18.7
1965	20.0	20.7	21.4	17.7	18.1	18.6
1964	20.1	21.0	21.5	17.2	17.8	18.5
1963	20.0	21.0	21.5	17.2	17.9	18.5
1962	20.0	21.0	21.5	---	---	18.6
1961	20.2	21.1	21.6	---	---	18.6
1960	20.2	21.3	21.8	17.2	17.9	18.4

In 1969 the teenage marriage rate, computed by relating the estimated number of marriages at ages under twenty years to the unmarried population fifteen to nineteen years of age, was 88 per 1,000 women, and 35 per 1,000 men.

A number of factors affect the incidence of teenage marriage in a particular state and variation among states within the same geographic division and region. Among them are state marriage laws and population composition by age, race, sex and religion.

To some extent teenage marriage occurs more frequently in states that are permissive in their standards regarding age at marriage. Of the states for which data on age at marriage were available in 1969, twenty had a relatively low legal minimum age for at least one partner. Of these twenty states, twelve had proportions of teenage marriages above the United States average of 33.4 for brides and 14.5 for grooms. These states were Kentucky, Alabama, North Carolina, South Carolina, Utah, Mississippi, Missouri, Tennessee, Texas, Oregon, Michigan and Georgia. All but three of the twelve states allowed females under sixteen years, males under eighteen, or both to marry with parental consent. (See Tables 3 and 4, and Figure 1.)

Table 3. Estimated number of teenage brides and grooms with percent change: United States and each geographic region, 1960 and 1969

[By area of occurrence]

Region	Bride			Groom		
	1969	1960	Percent change	1969	1960	Percent change
United States ...	717,000	557,000	+28.7	311,000	201,000	+54.7
Northeast	102,000	92,000	+10.9	38,000	29,000	+31.0
North Central	185,000	152,000	+21.7	83,000	58,000	+43.1
South	291,000	214,000	+36.0	131,000	77,000	+70.1
West	140,000	99,000	+41.4	59,000	38,000	+55.3

Table 4. Teenage marriage rates, by sex: United States and each geographic region, 1960
[By area of occurrence. Rates per 1,000 unmarried population in specified group.]

Region	Female	Male
United States	100.3	31.2
South	121.6	35.2
West	120.6	37.5
North Central	95.8	32.6
Northeast	66.2	19.5

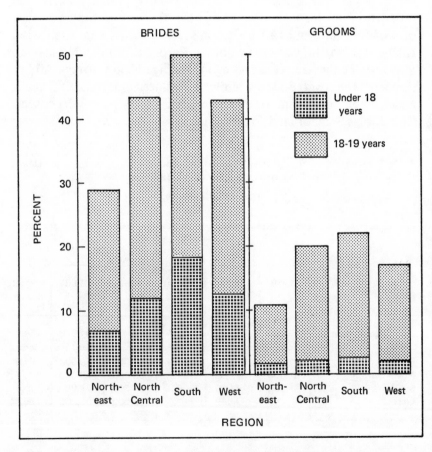

Figure 1. Percentage of first marriages involving teenage brides and grooms, by age: marriage-registration area states grouped by geographic region, 1969.

24

Legislation regarding age at marriage was revised or enacted in several states during the sixties. A review of the nature of these revisions showed changes in the number of teenagers married. Following a change in Iowa marriage law that raised the legal minimum age with parental consent, the number of teenagers married in that state fell from 15,020 in 1960 to 10,740 in 1962, the first full year after the change, a twenty-nine percent decline.

A change of even greater magnitude occurred in Idaho in 1967 after the law was revised to raise the legal minimum age with and without parental consent, and to establish a three-day waiting period. The number of teenagers married declined from 12,665 in 1966 to 5,020 in 1968, a sixty percent drop. Increases, though small, occurred in the adjoining states.

The opposite effect was produced in Kentucky when limits were relaxed for both partners in marriage without parental consent. The number of teenagers marrying rose from 18,030 in 1967 to 26,190 in 1969, a forty-five percent increase.

Effective in 1969, Texas lowered the age at which consent for males is required and dropped the three-day waiting period before issuance of a license. The number of brides and grooms under twenty marrying in Texas increased from 62,135 in 1968 to 79,863 in 1969 (an increase of twenty-nine percent). (See Figure 2 and Table 5.)

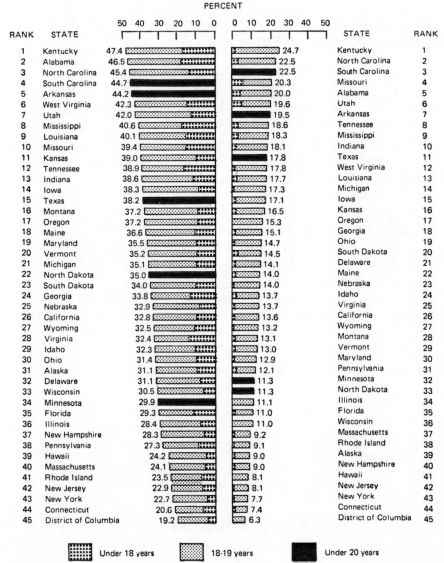

BRIDES   PERCENT   GROOMS

		50 40 30 20 10 0	0 10 20 30 40 50		
RANK	STATE			STATE	RANK
1	Kentucky	47.4	24.7	Kentucky	1
2	Alabama	46.5	22.5	North Carolina	2
3	North Carolina	45.4	22.5	South Carolina	3
4	South Carolina	44.7	20.3	Missouri	4
5	Arkansas	44.2	20.0	Alabama	5
6	West Virginia	42.3	19.6	Utah	6
7	Utah	42.0	19.5	Arkansas	7
8	Mississippi	40.6	18.6	Tennessee	8
9	Louisiana	40.1	18.3	Mississippi	9
10	Missouri	39.4	18.1	Indiana	10
11	Kansas	39.0	17.8	Texas	11
12	Tennessee	38.9	17.8	West Virginia	12
13	Indiana	38.6	17.7	Louisiana	13
14	Iowa	38.3	17.3	Michigan	14
15	Texas	38.2	17.1	Iowa	15
16	Montana	37.2	16.5	Kansas	16
17	Oregon	37.2	15.3	Oregon	17
18	Maine	36.6	15.1	Georgia	18
19	Maryland	35.5	14.7	Ohio	19
20	Vermont	35.2	14.5	South Dakota	20
21	Michigan	35.1	14.1	Delaware	21
22	North Dakota	35.0	14.0	Maine	22
23	South Dakota	34.0	14.0	Nebraska	23
24	Georgia	33.8	13.7	Idaho	24
25	Nebraska	32.9	13.7	Virginia	25
26	California	32.8	13.6	California	26
27	Wyoming	32.5	13.2	Wyoming	27
28	Virginia	32.4	13.1	Montana	28
29	Idaho	32.3	13.0	Vermont	29
30	Ohio	31.4	12.9	Maryland	30
31	Alaska	31.1	12.1	Pennsylvania	31
32	Delaware	31.1	11.3	Minnesota	32
33	Wisconsin	30.5	11.3	North Dakota	33
34	Minnesota	29.9	11.1	Illinois	34
35	Florida	29.3	11.0	Florida	35
36	Illinois	28.4	11.0	Wisconsin	36
37	New Hampshire	28.3	9.2	Massachusetts	37
38	Pennsylvania	27.3	9.1	Rhode Island	38
39	Hawaii	24.2	9.0	Alaska	39
40	Massachusetts	24.1	9.0	New Hampshire	40
41	Rhode Island	23.5	8.1	Hawaii	41
42	New Jersey	22.9	8.1	New Jersey	42
43	New York	22.7	7.7	New York	43
44	Connecticut	20.6	7.4	Connecticut	44
45	District of Columbia	19.2	6.3	District of Columbia	45

Under 18 years   18-19 years   Under 20 years

Figure 2: State rankings by percent of all marriages involving teenage brides and grooms, by age: 44 reporting states and the District of Columbia, 1969.

Table 5. Percent distribution of brides and grooms at specified ages by marriage order: marriage-registration area and each geographic region, 1969.

[By area of occurrence. Based on sample data]

Sex and age	Marriage-registration area	Region			
		Northeast	North Central[1]	South[2]	West[3]
Bride					
All marriages	100.0	100.0	100.0	100.0	100.0
Under 20 years	32.6	24.5	33.7	37.8	33.3
Under 18 years	9.8	6.0	9.2	13.5	9.4
18-19 years	22.8	18.4	24.4	24.3	23.9
20 years and over	67.4	75.6	66.3	62.2	66.7
First marriages	100.0	100.0	100.0	100.0	100.0
Under 20 years	41.4	29.0	43.3	49.9	43.1
Under 18 years	12.5	7.1	12.0	18.1	12.3
18-19 years	28.9	21.9	31.3	31.8	30.8
20 years and over	58.6	71.0	56.7	50.1	56.9
Groom					
All marriages	100.0	100.0	100.0	100.0	100.0
Under 20 years	13.9	9.2	15.2	16.7	13.7
Under 18 years	1.5	1.2	1.4	1.9	1.3
18-19 years	12.5	8.0	13.9	14.8	12.3
20 years and over	86.1	90.8	84.8	83.3	86.3
First marriages	100.0	100.0	100.0	100.0	100.0
Under 20 years	18.0	11.0	19.8	22.3	17.8
Under 18 years	1.9	1.4	1.7	2.5	1.8
18-19 years	16.1	9.7	18.1	19.8	16.1
20 years and over	82.0	89.0	80.2	77.7	82.2

[1] Excludes Minnesota and North Dakota.
[2] Excludes Arkansas, Oklahoma, Texas and South Carolina.
[3] Excludes Colorado, New Mexico, Arizona, Nevada and Washington.

27

Divorce Among Teenagers and Among Individuals Who Married During Their Teens

Concern over teenage marriage focuses on the stability of these unions and whether they are more likely to end in divorce than marriages contracted at older ages. In 1969 an estimated 28,000 teenage women and 6,000 teenage men were granted divorces. Expressed as divorce rates, approximately 28 out of every 1,000 teenage wives and 19 of every 1,000 teenage husbands were granted a divorce during that year.

Annual age-specific divorce rates, relating the number of divorces granted during a year by age at divorce to the married population of the same ages do not adequately reflect the instability of teenage marriages. A major consideration is the very short time a marriage is at risk of ending in divorce during teenage years. A person married at age nineteen scarcely has time to obtain a divorce while still a teenager. Since in most states the legal requirement alone results in lapses of at least several months, many relatively quick breakups of teenage marriages do not show up in the teenage divorce rate.

Data is available for twenty-one states. The Bureau of the Census reports that twenty-seven percent of the women with teenage marriages were known to have been divorced within twenty or more years, as compared with fourteen percent of those who entered first marriage after they had reached their twenties. Twenty-eight percent of those men who married before the age of twenty-two years were known to have been divorced, as compared with thirteen percent of those who married for the first time after they had reached twenty-two years of age. In other words, divorce was twice as likely for early marriages as for those contracted at later ages.

Persons who married before age twenty account for varying proportions of divorces from state to state, and regional differences are apparent in the figures in Table 6. As can be seen, in 1969 the highest proportion of such divorces was shown by the South, based on data from only three states of that region. The North Central and Northeast regions ranked second and third, and in the West persons who had married in their teens accounted for the smallest proportion of divorces granted during the year, giving the region a rank of fourth.

Table 6. Percentage of divorced husbands and wives who were teenagers at time of decree and percentage married when teenagers: divorce-registration area and 20 reporting states, grouped by region, 1969

[Based on sample data. By place of occurrence. Computed on totals excluding figures for age not stated]

Region and State	Divorced husbands who were teenagers at time of:		Divorced wives who were teenagers at time of:	
	Decree	Marriage	Decree	Marriage
	Percent			
Divorce-registration area[1]	0.9	19.2	4.4	45.8
Northeast - - - - - - - - - - - - - -	0.5	17.7	2.8	45.8
Vermont - - - - - - - - - - - - - - - - -	0.4	19.5	2.6	51.4
Rhode Island - - - - - - - - - - - - - -	0.3	16.3	2.1	44.8
Connecticut - - - - - - - - - - - - - -	0.2	15.2	1.9	42.1
New York - - - - - - - - - - - - - - - -	0.5	15.3	2.2	43.6
Pennsylvania - - - - - - - - - - - - - -	0.7	20.6	3.7	48.9
North Central - - - - - - - - - - - -	1.0	19.4	5.3	47.0
Illinois - - - - - - - - - - - - - - - - - -	0.8	17.6	4.5	45.1
Wisconsin - - - - - - - - - - - - - - -	0.3	16.9	2.0	48.1
Iowa - - - - - - - - - - - - - - - - - -	1.8	22.9	6.4	50.2
Missouri - - - - - - - - - - - - - - -	1.3	22.0	6.7	48.1
Nebraska - - - - - - - - - - - - - - -	0.8	17.3	5.6	46.2
Kansas - - - - - - - - - - - - - - -	1.7	21.8	7.3	49.5
South - - - - - - - - - - - - - -	1.6	25.1	7.1	52.5
Virginia - - - - - - - - - - - - - - - -	0.5	24.1	3.4	52.3
Kentucky - - - - - - - - - - - - - - -	1.8	25.7	9.2	52.4
Tennessee - - - - - - - - - - - - - -	2.2	25.5	8.8	52.7
West - - - - - - - - - - - - - - - - -	0.6	16.2	2.9	40.8
Montana - - - - - - - - - - - - - - -	1.3	12.7	6.2	41.2
Idaho - - - - - - - - - - - - - - - - - -	2.1	14.5	6.9	41.0
Oregon - - - - - - - - - - - - - - - -	1.0	16.9	4.1	44.0
California - - - - - - - - - - - - - - -	0.5	16.4	2.5	40.7
Alaska - - - - - - - - - - - - - - - -	0.3	13.5	4.3	41.5
Hawaii - - - - - - - - - - - - - - - -	0.1	13.2	2.1	34.7

[1]Includes cases for Alabama, Georgia, Maryland, Michigan, Ohio, South Dakota, Utah, and Wyoming, which are not shown separately.

29

As observed earlier, the South also accounted for the greatest proportion of teenage marriages. However, comparisons that may be made between marriage and divorce data by region are limited because data on divorces are not available for all states reporting marriage data. (Table 7 and Figure 3.)

Table 7. Estimated number and rate of divorces, by age at time of decree and sex: United States, 1969

[Rates per 1,000 married population in specified group]

Age	Female		Male	
	Number	Rate	Number	Rate
All ages - - -	639,000	13.4	639,000	13.8
Under 20 years - - -	27,900	28.2	5,800	19.0
20-24 years - - - - -	153,700	30.7	102,000	34.0
25-29 years - - - - -	136,200	24.3	139,800	27.7
30-34 years - - - - -	89,800	17.8	102,700	21.8
35-44 years - - - - -	136,900	13.1	154,900	15.5
45-54 years - - - - -	68,800	7.1	90,600	9.3
55-64 years - - - - -	20,200	3.1	32,100	4.3
65 years and over - - - - - - - -	5,500	1.4	11,200	1.9

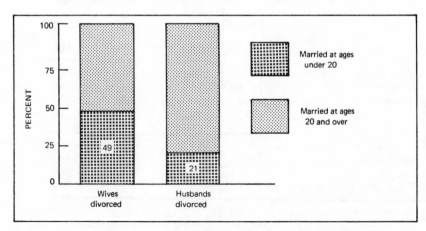

Figure 3. Percentage of husbands and wives divorced in 1969 who had married as teenagers; 21 reporting states.

Illegitimate Births

In 1968, while accounting for fourteen percent of legitimate births in the United States, teenage women accounted for forty-nine percent of illegitimate births. (See Figure 4.) The estimated 165,700 illegitimate births to teenage mothers that year were almost as many as were recorded for all other age groups of women combined. This count was about eighty percent above the number in 1960, a much greater increase than occurred in illegitimate births to women of all other ages (thirty-one percent). In contrast, legitimate births to teenagers were thirteen percent fewer than in 1960, a smaller decrease than the other women experienced (twenty-three percent).

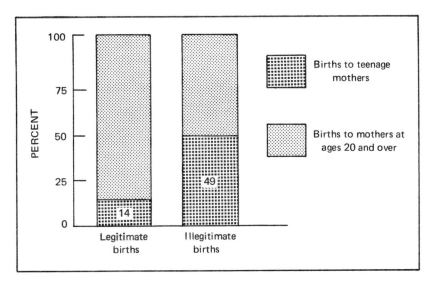

Figure 4. Percentage of births to teenage mothers by estimated legitimacy status: United States, 1968.

Illegitimate births accounted for a larger proportion of all births for teenage women than for women in any other age group. In 1968, an estimated 276 of every 1,000 births to women under twenty years of age were illegitimate, and the younger the teenage mother, the greater the likelihood of illegitimacy. At ages under fifteen years an estimated 810 of every 1,000 births were illegitimate, at ages fifteen to seventeen the ratio was 404 per 1,000, and at ages eighteen to nineteen it was 201 per 1,000. (Tables 8 and 9.)

Table 8. Estimated number and ratio of illegitimate births, by age of mother and color: United States, 1968

[Due to rounding estimates to the nearest hundred, figures by color may not add to totals. Ratios per 1,000 total live births in specified group]

Age	Number			Ratio		
	Total	White	All other	Total	White	All other
Total	339,200	155,200	183,900	96.9	53.3	312.0
Under 15 years	7,700	1,900	5,800	810.2	610.1	907.7
15-19 years	158,000	67,400	90,600	267.2	158.0	549.7
15-17 years	77,900	28,400	49,400	403.7	234.4	688.0
18-19 years	80,100	39,000	41,200	201.1	127.7	443.0
20-24 years	107,900	56,800	51,100	82.6	51.0	264.0
25-29 years	35,200	16,100	19,100	38.9	20.4	168.0
30-34 years	17,200	7,300	10,000	41.0	20.5	155.3
35-39 years	9,700	4,200	5,500	47.1	24.5	157.2
40 years and over	3,300	1,500	1,800	51.4	28.4	156.5

Table 9. Marital status of population and legitimacy status of births for females at ages 15-19 and 20-24: United States, 1968

Status	Age of females	
	15-19 years	20-24 years
Population		
Total	8,949,000	7,809,000
Married	952,000	4,818,000
Unmarried	7,997,000	2,991,000
Births		
Total	591,312	1,306,872
Legitimate	433,312	1,198,972
Illegitimate	158,000	107,900

Another important factor was the proportion of illegitimate live births. This increased for teenage mothers throughout the sixties. From 1960 to 1968 the increase in the proportion of illegitimate births was greater for teenage mothers than for mothers in any other age group. The increase for teenagers was least at age fifteen and more for each subsequent single year of age, being greatest at age nineteen, where the proportion almost doubled. (Figure 5.)

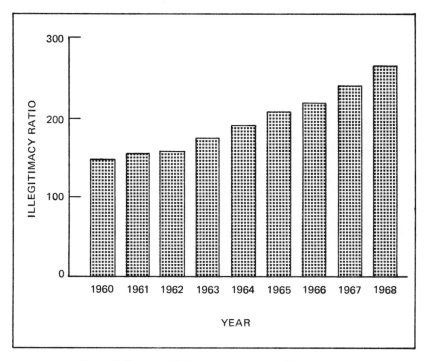

Figure 5. Estimated illegitimacy ratios per 1,000 live births
for births to mothers aged 15-19: United States, 1960-68.

Infants born to teenage mothers face greater risks of death or deformity than infants born to women at older ages. The infant mortality rate in the United States, which has not been brought down to the low levels attained by a number of economically and medically advanced Western European countries, has been looked upon with concern in recent years. In the search for possible causes, it has been noted that risk of death is greatest for infants physically underdeveloped at time of birth and that the percentage of births in this category is greatest for births to very young mothers.

In the United States, the risk of death in the first year of life among infants who weighed 2,500 grams or less at birth was found to be seventeen times the risk among infants weighing more. In addition to the greater risk of death, there was greater prevalence among infants with low birth weight of such conditions as cerebral palsy, epilepsy, mental retardation, congenital anomalies, deafness and blindness. Infants born to teenage mothers are more likely to be of low birth weight than infants born to older mothers. The proportion of infants weighing 2,500 grams or less at birth was highest among mothers at the youngest ages.[4]

Venereal Disease

According to McKesson Laboratories in their booklet "Venereal Disease–America's Modern Plague," the number of cases of venereal disease *that were reported* was shockingly higher in 1970 than in 1957.

In 1957, there were 6,251 cases of syphilis reported, and 20,168 cases in 1970. In 1957 there were 216,476 cases of gonorrhea reported, while in 1970 the number had increased to 573,200.

It is estimated that *less than one case of syphilis in four is reported.* This means that over 6,200 *new* cases develop *each month,* or more than 75,000 cases of infectious syphilis develop each year. Over 2,000,000 cases of infectious gonorrhea are caught by persons in the United States each year.

There are nearly 5,600 new cases of venereal disease caught *every day,* and over 1,300 of these are in teenagers. The rate among teenagers is more than two and a half times the rate of all age groups.

---

[4]Data from the National Vital Statistics System, "Vital and Health Statistics," Series Number 23–"Teenagers, Divorces, Parenthood, and Mortality," DHEW Publication No. (H.R.A.) 74-1901, August 1973.

On the basis of research conducted in Macon County, Alabama, it has been estimated that the life expectancy of a male between the ages of twenty-five and sixty years, infected with syphilis and receiving no treatment for his infection, is reduced by about seventeen percent.

During 1967, over 2,300 Americans died of syphilis. Many others became blind, deaf, insane, sterile or otherwise incapacitated.

Premarital tests in twenty-seven states uncovered 12,250 persons who were serologically positive for syphilis. One out of every eighty-one marriage applicants had laboratory evidence of syphilis. Most of these persons are immediately treated to prevent spread of venereal disease to their partner.

Table 10 gives the statistics in terms of states for the years 1971 and 1972.

TABLE 10(A). Newly Reported Civilian Cases of Venereal Diseases and Rates per 100,000 Population, United States by Geographic Division, 1971 and 1972.

AREA	SYPHILIS PRIMARY/SECONDARY Cases 1972	Cases 1971	Rates 1972	SYPHILIS ALL STAGES Cases 1972	Rates 1972	GONORRHEA Cases 1972	Cases 1971	Rates 1972	OTHER VENEREAL[1] DISEASES Cases 1972
U.S. TOTAL[2]	24,429	23,783	11.8	91,149	44.2	767,215	670,268	371.6	2,251
NEW ENGLAND	882	621	7.3	2,949	24.5	21,894	19,922	182.2	16
Maine	29	14	2.9	102	10.0	996	974	97.9	–
New Hampshire	10	5	1.3	61	8.0	662	559	86.3	1
Vermont	18	5	3.9	68	14.7	506	413	109.5	–
Massachusetts	517	317	9.0	1,830	31.7	10,307	9,942	178.8	12
Rhode Island	35	41	3.7	187	20.0	1,572	1,259	167.8	1
Connecticut	273	239	8.9	701	22.9	7,851	6,775	256.2	2
MIDDLE ATLANTIC	5,959	5,646	15.9	19,786	52.7	102,303	83,920	272.3	156
New York	4,475	4,300	24.4	11,746	64.1	64,882	55,174	353.8	90
New Jersey	942	945	12.9	3,768	51.5	16,676	11,485	227.8	23
Pennsylvania	542	401	4.5	4,272	35.9	20,745	17,261	174.1	43
EAST NORTH CENTRAL	2,596	2,731	6.4	16,761	41.0	118,243	115,958	289.5	371
Ohio	315	461	2.9	2,819	26.2	29,680	29,689	275.6	71
Indiana	265	330	5.0	1,101	20.8	11,318	8,621	214.2	3
Illinois	1,191	1,028	10.6	7,083	63.2	44,664	48,054	398.4	116
Michigan	763	853	8.4	4,890	53.9	24,749	22,270	273.0	180
Wisconsin	62	59	1.4	868	19.2	7,832	7,324	173.4	1
WEST NORTH CENTRAL	291	412	2.3	5,453	43.1	46,426	42,148	367.3	58
Minnesota	65	71	1.7	420	10.8	8,347	6,221	214.4	2
Iowa	52	23	1.8	487	16.9	6,187	6,115	214.7	12
Missouri	108	231	2.3	3,191	67.5	17,065	16,216	361.2	37
North Dakota	2	6	.3	18	2.9	686	626	110.6	–
South Dakota	2	9	.3	19	2.8	1,477	1,540	219.5	1
Nebraska	19	24	1.3	230	15.2	4,505	4,428	297.8	1

SOUTH ATLANTIC[2]	6,496	5,789	20.8	18,423	59.0	178,056	140,459	570.3	1,160
Delaware	59	35	10.6	160	28.6	2,139	1,640	382.6	1
Maryland	797	652	19.9	2,975	74.5	15,526	14,669	388.6	9
Virginia	594	348	12.9	2,221	48.2	16,887	15,487	366.8	31
West Virginia	34	32	1.9	868	48.8	1,953	1,904	109.7	2
North Carolina	545	444	10.6	1,476	28.8	25,088	20,565	489.9	80
South Carolina	502	404	19.3	1,171	45.1	25,532	15,524	983.1	88
Georgia	1,411	1,585	30.2	3,542	75.9	32,199	28,484	690.2	304
Florida	1,680	1,675	23.5	3,691	51.5	43,033	30,665	600.8	274
EAST SOUTH CENTRAL	1,536	1,273	11.8	3,317	25.5	61,721	47,223	474.5	130
Kentucky	398	331	12.2	1,152	35.3	7,825	6,767	239.4	11
Tennessee	514	367	12.8	1,047	26.1	26,592	20,546	662.6	53
Alabama	217	175	6.2	392	11.2	15,593	10,547	447.3	6
Mississippi	407	400	18.2	726	32.4	11,711	9,363	522.6	60
WEST SOUTH CENTRAL	2,924	3,555	14.8	9,768	49.4	93,799	79,625	474.5	210
Arkansas	174	247	8.8	946	48.0	10,707	7,949	543.8	6
Louisiana	845	747	22.9	2,191	59.5	16,306	13,916	442.5	116
Oklahoma	104	105	4.0	1,118	42.9	9,539	7,567	365.9	11
Texas	1,801	2,456	15.7	5,513	48.0	57,247	50,193	498.0	77
MOUNTAIN	528	590	6.1	1,963	22.5	23,566	19,949	270.4	33
Montana	7	1	1.0	21	2.9	1,368	1,136	191.9	5
Idaho	8	12	1.1	16	2.1	1,998	1,721	266.0	2
Wyoming	13	3	3.8	72	21.1	421	239	123.5	–
Colorado	98	73	4.2	366	15.8	6,343	5,618	274.1	1
New Mexico	105	157	10.0	459	43.7	4,164	2,833	396.6	15
Arizona	198	215	10.3	689	36.0	5,720	5,325	298.7	8
Utah	20	15	1.8	158	14.1	1,590	1,232	141.8	–
Nevada	79	114	15.2	182	35.1	1,962	1,845	378.0	2
PACIFIC	3,217	3,166	12.0	12,729	47.5	121,207	121,064	452.7	117
Washington	129	142	3.8	304	8.9	11,033	9,293	323.9	8
Oregon	40	15	1.8	113	5.2	10,206	9,030	468.4	2
California	3,006	2,971	14.9	12,135	60.3	96,309	98,530	478.4	107
Alaska	12	17	4.0	91	30.5	2,098	2,540	704.0	–
Hawaii	30	21	4.0	86	11.3	1,561	1,671	205.7	–
Puerto Rico	796	824	28.7	2,143	28.7	2,506	2,141	90.2	1
Virgin Islands	89	29	156.1	394	691.2	588	607	1031.6	1

[1]U.S. total consists of cases of chancroid, cases of granuloma inguinale and cases of lymphogranuloma venereum.
[2]Includes cases reported by District of Columbia.

Data from the National Vital Statistics System, *Morbidity and Mortality Weekly Report. Annual Supplement 1972.*

TABLE 10(B). Newly Reported Civilian Cases of Venereal Diseases and Rates per 100,000 Population: United States by Age* and Sex, 1971 and 1972

Primary and Secondary Syphilis—1972

Age Group	Male Cases	Male Rates	Female Cases	Female Rates	Total Cases	Total Rates
0-14	92	.3	231	.8	323	.6
15-19	1,883	19.0	2,047	20.7	3,930	19.9
20-24	4,509	55.4	2,603	28.9	7,112	41.5
25-29	3,452	48.5	1,407	18.6	4,859	33.1
30-34	2,536	43.4	837	13.4	3,373	27.9
35-39	1,461	27.9	425	7.5	1,886	17.3
40-44	1,018	18.2	282	4.7	1,300	11.3
45-49	567	9.8	156	2.5	723	6.0
50 & over	774	3.3	149	.5	923	1.8
TOTAL	16,292	16.3	8,137	7.6	24,429	11.8

Gonorrhea—1972

Age Group	Male Cases	Male Rates	Female Cases	Female Rates	Total Cases	Total Rates
0-14	2,929	10.1	7,420	26.7	10,349	18.2
15-19	104,754	1058.2	97,403	987.3	202,157	1022.8
20-24	210,908	2593.2	101,167	1121.7	312,075	1819.5
25-29	99,498	1398.6	33,257	440.0	132,755	904.8
30-34	41,630	712.1	11,957	192.0	53,587	443.9
35-39	21,183	404.1	5,605	98.9	26,788	245.5
40-44	11,417	204.5	2,814	47.2	14,231	123.3
45-49	6,217	107.9	1,363	21.9	7,580	63.2
50 & over	6,039	26.0	1,654	5.8	7,693	14.9
TOTAL	504,575	506.1	262,640	246.0	767,215	371.6

Congenital Syphilis—1971-1972

Age Group	Number of Cases 1971	Number of Cases 1972	Percent of Total 1971	Percent of Total 1972
0-1	452	383	22.0	21.8
1-4	58	16	2.8	0.9
5-9	30	11	1.5	0.6
10+	1,512	1,348	73.7	76.7
TOTAL	2,052	1,758	100.0	100.0

*Age data for 1972—provisional

38

Local Information

Check with your local Department of Health for information relative to your community.

Occasionally you will find articles in your local newspaper such as the following one. It can certainly help to make your case stronger when presented to the school board and to the parents and members of the community.

Increase in Island VD rate more than double rest of nation

By LEONARD BALDASSANO

The increase of venereal disease on Staten Island has soared ahead of the rest of the nation as Island Health Department officials report the number of people treated, mostly college age, has nearly tripled since 1971.

Wayne Olinzock, public health advisor for the VD clinic at the Richmond Health Center, gave the figures as 633 treated last year as compared with 430 in 1972 and 239 in 1971. But rather than finding these statistics disturbing he said:

"Actually I'm very gratified. It's an indication the program is working and we are getting the message across. However we haven't been seeing as many high school students as before .. for some reason they don't think they can catch it."

To spread the message the Island Health Department is waging an intensive campaign, particularly in high schools, with posters, films and lectures.

"It's part of an overall city-wide campaign aimed at doing a projected 750,000 cultures this year," Olinzock said, adding that infectious syphilis and gonorrhea know no social or economic bounds.

Although figures on the Island are still proportionally low per 100,000 people the rate of gonorrhea from 1971-72 has increased by 25.4 per cent as compared with 13.8 per cent in the city and 11.1 per cent in the nation, Bureau of Statistics figures show.

Infectious syphilis has slightly decreased in the city by 10.2 per cent and 4.3 per cent in the nation while Island figures leveled off with the number of cases treated in 1971 equaling those in 1972. Statistics for 1973 were not available.

According to Olinzock, there are no accurate statistics on which to base comparisons although he pointed out the national upward trend of venereal disease represented a true pandemic.

The actual number of cases on the Island may be more numerous than reported, according to health department officials, because many private physicians rarely report the incidence of the disease among their patients. An American Health Association survey estimates that only one physician in 10 reports his cases to health clinics.

Dr. Patricia A. Nolan, regional health director for Richmond stressed the importance of receiving reports of all VD cases from private physicians. Failure to report, she said, hampers health department investigators in controlling the disease by concealing the contacts that harbor the infectious germ cells.

"The cases that aren't reported, possibly for confidentiality, don't allow public health advisers to follow up and contact those people who are continuing to spread the disease," Nolan said.

Other variables adding to the inaccurate count of VD on the Island is the number of Islanders attending night clinics in the city. If these cases were figured in with Island statistics, Olinzock said, the incidence of reported VD would be considerably larger.

Besides Staten Island's city clinic, 25 Stuyvesant Place, St. George, which is open weekly: Tuesdays from 9 a.m. to 11 a.m. and Thursdays from 1 p.m. to 3 p.m., there are four other clinics that screen for VD.

Richmond and Staten Island Community Colleges receive materials from the Department of Health for routine gonorrhea screenings requested by the students.

The Staten Island Community Corporation Family and Planning Health Clinic at 1195 Castleton Ave., West Brighton, administers free gonorrhea screenings to all male patients. It is open on Monday and Thursday mornings and on Monday and Wednesday evenings.

Staten Island Hospital gives gonorrhea screenings to female patients strictly by appointment.

Children and Youth Receive Most Sex Education from Their Peers, Not Their Parents

Most people have to go no further than their own experiences to verify this statement. We ask you, "Where did you personally get most of your sex information? Where did you turn, when there was something of a sexual nature you were curious about?" No statistics we know of are available for this, but until recent years most young people, while growing up, consulted their peers, and sometimes older brothers or sisters (usually a sibling of the same sex). The author recalls trying to find out, at the age of fourteen, what an abortion was. Friends were consulted who didn't know either, and next the dictionary was used. It gave the meaning as "a miscarriage." This definition didn't satisfy us either. As a last resort we went to the mother of one of the girls. She told us, but it was an embarrassing situation of the greatest magnitude, and one we never repeated.

In our time, young people received much information from the media, but the discussion of it, for many, many of them, was reserved for their friends. In schools where sex education is being taught, this is changing. Where the teacher has been able to establish a climate of "trust, not tryst," sex information is regarded far more casually than before.

When young people receive information from their peers it is often inaccurate, and given with overtones of secrecy and anxiety. So-called facts are often couched in a framework of the utmost confusion. The entire subject of masturbation is an example of this. When children receive their sex education from other children, guilt often accompanies any sex interest or urge. How many children have any concept of the effect these guilt feelings can have on them in later life?

Many young people will seek information in books—but so often books of the lurid-cover variety. The magazines they peruse are also sources of their sex education. The question of moral values may never, ever be brought to their attention.

Our children are constantly asked to make decisions in terms of experimentation in sexual activity as well as in the areas of drugs, alcohol, even crime. When they turn to their peers for assistance, it is often the blind leading the blind. Or, even more serious to comtemplate, it may be a situation in which misery wants company, and a child with guilt feelings encourages his or her friends to experiment and join the crowd. Peers are sometimes able to give advice to their friends, but is this the advice we want them to get?

Concerned Parents Feel a Strong Need for Providing Sex Education

Many parents are in revolt today against the cheap image that sex has taken in our society today. One look at movie advertisements is enough to illustrate this image. Furthermore, young children often do gain admittance to such movies. We have seen youngsters standing in front of such theaters—and even if they don't get in, there are still photographs exhibited. What was once considered pornography is now commonplace. Television shows are becoming more and more unrestricted, as far as the image of sex is concerned. So-called family shows can be embarrassing to adults as well as to the youngsters viewing them.

Many concerned parents are not convinced that they can do the whole job of providing accurate, factual information about human growth and development. Many parents even question whether or not they are the best source for objective learning of sex information, especially for their teenagers. Most parents agree that the school can provide supplemental help in developing moral and ethical values concerning sex attitudes and conduct due to an objective environment for learning.

We strongly believe that any parent who does not wish his or her children to be given sex education should have these wishes respected. For the children of those parents who feel that they or their church are adequately teaching the youngsters, instruction in an alternate subject area should certainly be provided. Nor should such children be made to feel they are in any way different from the other children. This is purely a case of different philosophies, and in this, as in all areas, every person has a right to be respected. Since children are sensitive in such matters, this must be handled extremely tactfully, and the youngster involved not made to feel like an outcast.

The Sex Education Program Should Give Your Children the Specific Information They Want and Need to Know

In our era of struggle for relevancy in education, sex education is one of the most relevant of all subject areas. We must take into account many factors in regard to it.

1. *Not all individuals develop at the same rate—psychologically or physically.* In all teaching of this subject this must be considered. We can't rush the youngsters.

This brings to mind a well-known anecdote. Little Johnny,

aged seven, came in from outdoor play one late afternoon. "Mommy," he said, "Where do I come from?"

His mother has been waiting for this opportunity. She sat Johnny down, and began to describe the father and the sperm, the mother and the egg. She had just completed the bit about the egg when Johnny interrupted her.

"No, no, Mommy," he announced. "Billy just moved here. He comes from Pittsburgh. Where do I come from?"

Children must be ready for what is being taught to them. Shakespeare's phrase "The readiness is all" is so true in this respect.

2. No child should ever feel ill at ease about asking questions of his or her teacher or of his or her parents. An effective sex education teacher should be able to break down the barriers between child and teacher, and between child and parent. When sex education is treated as a school subject, just as science or social studies is treated, it puts a different light on it. It must be handled as a relative of both of those subject areas, as it surely is. Much of what is included in the curriculum is biology—anatomy and physiology. Some parents will recognize certain aspects from their studies of those courses. Then, from the social studies we have some topics, for example, psychology and mental hygiene. The strength of your program will depend on how much scientific information can be transmitted, but even more so on how the youngsters' attitudes will be formed. Family living is certainly the most vital of the topics we should teach in social studies.

3. Your sex education program should cover the subjects your parents want their children to know—covering them, of course, at the children's level of comprehension. There is no point in instituting a program from which many children will have to be excluded because parents want the children removed. While consensus is often difficult to obtain, it is vital that you attempt it.

The Sex Education Program in the Schools Should Provide an Opportunity to Reach Parents and Assist Them with Their Questions

There are few parents who are professional educators. Those who are rarely have at their finger tips a full program in any subject area. Nor do they have textbooks and audio-visual aids at their disposal. Even teachers not prepared specifically for teaching sex education would have difficulty. Sex education is a highly organized, specific body of information, developed to meet the needs of children and their parents.

Furthermore, many parents are products of a generation when formal sex education was not provided. They admit to being confused about the facts of human growth and reproduction. Some reveal that they hold irrational fears and superstitions about sexual conduct that has been carried over since childhood. In some communities, courses in sex education and/or family life have led to the establishment of courses or workshops for parents to assist them in this area by building up their backgrounds in technical terms and in organized subject matter.

The teacher selected for teaching sex education must be a very special type of person who relates well to both young people and parents. When necessary, he or she must be able to work with mothers and/or fathers in workshop situations or in small group or individual discussions.

As will be discussed, parents should be kept informed of the exact material being covered in their youngsters' classes. By giving them this information in advance, possible complications and disagreements may be avoided. A close rapport with the teacher is eminently desired. Parental previewing of both printed and audio-visual material is strongly recommended for two reasons. One is to gain their approval, or determine what to do if there is disapproval. Second is to give the parents the chance to discuss intelligently with the child what he or she is learning. Parents must be considered partners in this particular subject area.

Summary

We have stated a number of points that we feel will help you to gain acceptance for launching a sex education program. The statistics are tremendously important, for they show the need in the most obvious terms. The fact that children generally receive most of their sex education from the media and their peers, and that their education is at best incomplete and at worst confusing and misinforming, must certainly be taken into consideration.

Concerned parents in many communities, and possibly in yours, have realized the need for providing sex education in an objective, educational environment. Young people, too, realize this need, and many are seeking accurate information concerning normal development. The goals of your sex education program must include as top priority giving your children the specific information they want and need to know, and it should provide an opportunity to reach parents and assist them with their questions.

CHAPTER 2   *How to Organize*
and Develop the
Sex Education Program

Experience indicates that the development of a local family life and sex education program may require anywhere from two to four years. This time allotment is based on information gathered from schools that have gone through the process.

The material that follows was derived from the publication of the Illinois Sex Education Advisory Board, *Steps Toward Implementing Family Life and Sex Education Programs in Illinois Schools.* It was sent to us by Superintendent Michael J. Bakalis, Superintendent of Public Instruction. The information contained in this report was prepared for local school districts in Illinois that were in the process of, or considering, the establishment of sex education and family living programs. We feel it may be applicable to your situation.

The following items are proposed as logical steps in organizing a family life and sex education program. The points will be listed briefly and then discussed in some detail.

(1) Development of Initial Interest.
(2) Establishment of an Informal Exploratory Committee.
(3) Establishment of a Community Planning Committee.
(4) Formation of a Curriculum Committee.

(5) Approval by the Board of Education.
(6) Development of a Program of In-Service Training for Teachers.
(7) Initiation of the Program.

Initial Interest

Initial interest in sex education can originate from many sources both within and outside the school. Obviously, this interest is extremely important as it gives a realistic starting point rather than an artificial one. From experience, it is known that interest in sex education has arisen from physicians, teachers, students, parents, church groups, parent-teacher groups, the communications media and other groups. Frequently, the focus of interest is centered in a very small group who by discussing the topic with other people will find that there are many persons with a genuine interest in sex education. Many authorities feel that it is a healthy situation when the initial interest for developing sex education programs develops, in part, outside the school.

Informal Exploratory Committee

Following initial interest, the usual procedure is that the persons who are most interested in sex education will organize a small (twelve members or less) informal exploratory committee that will study sex education further and will determine a course of action to follow. The main concern of this committee should be to convey its findings to the appropriate authorities.

In most situations the recommendations of this committee will be conveyed to the school administration. It is usually the responsibility of the administrative officials to recommend that the third step be taken.

This committee can usually complete its work in three months or less.

Community Planning Committee

The procedure of establishing a school-community committee that will study the entire area of family life and sex education is most crucial and important. The primary responsibility of this committee should be to determine if a need exists for a family life and sex education program in the local community. The committee that is established should have the broadest possible representation from the community. It should not be overweighed with teachers and school personnel. All committees should have representation from the school administration, teachers, school nurses, parents, clergy of various faiths, the medical society, the parent-teacher groups and other community agencies that are interested in family health. Mental health, public health, and child and family services of all types should be included, and it is most important that the communications media have representation on the committee. The communications representatives can provide a continuous feedback to the community through their particular news medium, whether it be newspaper, radio or television.

It is important that the students for whom the family life and sex education program is being planned have an opportunity to make their feelings and interests known. Some school districts have included student representatives on the community planning committee. Other school districts have organized a committee of students to work in conjunction with the community planning committee. When such a committee is formed, representatives should report to the community planning committee at appropriate intervals. School districts should not overlook the important contributions that students will make if encouraged to do so.

The community planning committee will deal with the wide variety of problems that are associated with the community. Almost all communities in taking a sober look at human sexuality and sex education will find many problems. Typical problems have received wide exposure in the past ten years. Venereal disease, illegitimate births, abortion, unmarried pregnant teenagers, divorce, broken homes, family disintegration and misconceptions about human sexuality are widespread in contemporary society. The committee should also deal with such questions as: What is sex education? What do we expect a program in sex education to accomplish? When should it start? What types of experiences should be provided for youngsters? What are the feelings of various interested groups such as the ministerial society, medical society and other groups involved in the welfare of youth toward programs in family life and sex education?

This committee should also concern itself with methods and procedures for interpreting to the community what the committee is attempting to do. Many people look upon sex education as mainly reproductive education; this is unfortunate. One of the early factors that the committee is usually able to determine is that family life and sex education include much more than reproductive education. The long-range goal of a sex education program should be to help students to become more responsible adults with acceptable values and standards. It should also strengthen a student's sense of moral and ethical responsibility not only to himself but to his fellowman. It is equally important that youth understand the desirable benefits that accrue to our society through stable family life.

What is a desirable size for this committee? Usually communities in their earnest efforts to include every possible interested individual and group will end up with a committee of forty or fifty members. Such a group is much too large to function effectively. Committees of twenty members or less function better. It is important that there be a continuous interchange of ideas among individual members of the committee, and for this reason it is desirable to keep the committee within reasonable, manageable limits.

In studying these local ramifications this committee will encounter many problems. Some of these problems will be new to committee members. Usually, such committees will decide that there is a very definite need for a program in family life and sex education in their schools and communities.

In attempting to get community support for the program, many people will ask if a program of family life and sex education will alleviate the many problems that the committee has discovered through its study. At this point, committees should be very, very cautious. In their enthusiasm to gain support for a program, they are apt to promise all sorts of appealing, immediate results. The family life and sex education program is not going to prove to be an immediate panacea for all the community sexual-social ills. However, a strong program on family life and sex education should have a beneficial effect upon many social problems over a long period of time.

How long a period of time will the community planning committee need to complete its work? This is an exceedingly important question, but a very difficult one to answer. It is impossible to project a specific timetable that will work in all situations. Obviously, the personnel of the committee will determine the procedures to follow; these procedures will largely establish the amount of time required to complete the work.

The committee should not work so hastily that it fails to deal with all important aspects of the problem. Conversely, if the committee work is uninspired, sporadic and conducted over a long period of time, it is almost a certainty that interest and enthusiasm will wane and productiveness will be affected. Also, when committee work is extended beyond a reasonable period of time, there may be changes in personnel. This disturbs the rapport of the committee and requires that new committee members be brought up to date. Personnel changes should be avoided if at all possible.

Community planning committees have worked for varying periods of time. The time required may range from three months to two years. It seems reasonable to expect that the committee should be able to complete its work in six to nine months, rarely more than a year.

It is important that the committee, at its organizational meeting, set anticipated goals and a time schedule that will allow it to do a competent and thorough job.[1]

The state of Iowa, in its policy statement, suggests a different procedure, which follows.

I. Introducing the Program

   A. Initial Impetus

      1. School personnel may provide the impetus for encouraging the development of the program.
      2. Individuals or lay groups within the district may provide

------

[1] *Steps Toward Implementing Family Life and Sex Education Programs in Illinois Schools.* Used by permission.

the impetus for encouraging the development of the
program.

3. No matter what the impetus, the interest should be
   reported to the school administrators, who should decide
   what priority is to be given to the development of a
   program.

B. Administrative Follow-through

1. The superintendent should discuss the need for a program
   with the administrative staff.
2. The administration and teachers should determine what is
   already being done in the school in sex education, even
   though a structured program is not evident.
3. The administration should discuss the feasibility of such
   an addition to the curriculum with the board of education.

   The board of education and administration need to
   decide if a school staff committee should plan and
   promote the program, or if a lay advisory committee
   should be used. A lay advisory committee may be helpful.

   The board of education should place in its minutes the
   approval of the organizing of a committee to develop a
   program.

   Thereafter, the administration should keep the board of
   education informed on the progress or development of the
   program.

   A staff member should be appointed as committee
   chairman.
4. Reports and action concerning the program should be
   made available to interested groups.

It will be up to you, as the administrator, or to circum-
stances, to decide which path you wish to follow. Either one is
effective.

Parental Involvement

We feel that, as soon as the community planning committee has completed its work, the parents should be consulted. First, the study presented by the community planning committee should be submitted to the parent body, and discussed at great length. It is suggested that parents be elected to sit on the curriculum committee to insure that their viewpoint is constantly kept in mind. (You will note that parents were also on the community planning committee.)

You may wish to send a questionnaire to all parents, seeking their opinions. Almost all communities have some citizens, and schools some parents, who are opposed to the program. Some methods must be devised to take their wishes into consideration. It is also a well-known fact that, once a community has attempted to initiate a sex education program and has failed, it is usually many years before local boards of education, school officials, and citizens are interested in pursuing the project again.[2]

Making a Study to Determine the Type of Program the Parents Will Endorse

To gain information in regard to the parents' ideas in this area, you can hold discussions at parent meetings. Some suggested topics from the Iowa Statement of Objectives are:

1. What is an adequate definition of sex education?
2. Whose responsibility is sex education?
3. When should sex education begin?
4. Should sex education be a separate course? Should it be integrated with one or more existing curricula such as science, health, physical education or social studies?

[2]*Steps Toward Implementing Family Life and Sex Education Programs in Illinois Schools,* p. 11.

5. Who should teach the course?

6. How should the community be involved and informed to support the school program?

7. What should be included in a planned course for sex education and at what grade or age levels?

8. What is already being done by the church, school, home and community?

9. What is an appropriate title for the course? Sex Education? Health and Human Development? Family Life Education?

10. What are the objectives of the program?

11. How are the moral values taught along with the physiology of sex?

12. Should parents be given the option of having their children excused from the program?

13. What objections to the program are likely to arise?

14. Should boys and girls be taught together? At what grade levels?

At each subsequent meeting it is suggested that the committee of the whole preview films, sets of slides and filmstrips to determine what audiovisual aids are available for the K–12 sequential program and to make recommendations as to grade placement of the instructional materials.[3]

How to Establish the Objectives That Will Meet the Needs of Your Students

In order to have an idea of where your sex education program should be going, we have listed a series of objectives suggested by the Iowa State Board of Public Instruction. You may discover that they suit your needs (perhaps only temporarily) or you may find that you wish to change them. They are, however, a starting point from which you may move ahead.

---

[3]Iowa State Board of Public Instruction, Iowa *Statement of Objectives.* Used by permission.

You may wish to consult the parents or, having already learned their opinions, you may decide to turn this over to the curriculum committee.

The following objectives may supply the basis for your sex education program:

1. To provide the individual with adequate information about his own physical, mental and emotional maturation processes as related to sex.
2. To alleviate fears and anxieties relative to individual sexual development.
3. To develop objective and understanding attitudes toward sex in all of its various manifestations in the individual, toward himself, and toward others.
4. To give the individual insight concerning his relationships to members of both sexes and to help him understand his obligations and responsibilities to others.
5. To provide enough information about the misuses and deviations of sex as to enable the individual to protect himself against exploitation and against injury to his physical and mental health.
6. To provide a climate for the learning and the understanding that will enable each individual to utilize his sexuality effectively and creatively in his several roles, i.e., as a child, youth, spouse, parent, community member and citizen.
7. To build an understanding of the need for and appreciation of moral and ethical values that are necessary to provide a rational basis for making decisions concerning *all* human behavior.
8. To provide information as to the place of the family in our society and the skills that lead to a responsible home and family life.
9. To provide information and guidance about the emerging social problems that affect family in our society such as birth control and the population explosion, illegitimacy, early

marriage, venereal disease, solo parenthood, divorce and sexual deviation.

The Work of the Curriculum Committee

The establishment of a curriculum committee sanctioned by the board of education, which will ultimately develop curricular materials, is an important step. This committee should have a strong school orientation, since educators know curriculum construction and understand the educational process. This does not preclude, however, the contributions of competent resource people who may meet with the committee from time to time when their help is needed. Many school districts have used the services of physicians, psychiatrists, psychologists, social workers, sociologists, ministers, health educators and representatives of other disciplines effectively in developing curricular materials.

The curriculum committee will probably follow a rather typical pattern in working toward its ultimate goal. It will invariably go through a period of intense frustration, and even though this frustration is time-consuming and often very painful to the individuals involved, it seems a necessary step.

The typical committee will write to school districts in other states for materials that have been developed for local use in the hope that it can find a school system that has developed materials that can be adapted to meet the needs of the local district. Invariably, the final outcome is the same. After the committee has thoroughly examined the resource material that it has secured from other sources, it will probably reach the conclusion that none of the programs are specifically suited to the needs of the local school district. This leaves the committee, then, with the rather formidable task of developing materials for local use. The study of other districts' activities is an invaluable part of committee work and should be encouraged.[4]

---

[4]*Steps Toward Implementing Family Life and Sex Education Programs in Illinois Schools*, p. 15.

Again, it seems necessary to point out that communities vary considerably in their attitudes toward sex education. Materials that are accepted in one community may not be accepted in another.

Often, the individuals serving on this committee are uncomfortable when discussing sex education. Several school districts have thought it would be quite easy to employ a group of teachers for a summer session to construct a curriculum and have it ready for use by the opening of school that fall. These school districts, without exception, were amazed to find that it took six of the eight weeks before the teachers—people who had been working together for years—were able to talk with confidence and without embarrassment about sex education. This, again, is a needed part of the painful process of curriculum construction.

As soon as the curriculum committee gets some sense of direction, it should share its thinking with citizens of the community. For example, if particular films are recommended for showing at selected grade levels, these films should be shown to wide groups of parents in order to get their reactions to them. The more information that can be given to community citizens while the program is being developed, the better. In those situations where good channels of communication have been established within the community, most school districts have found that a high percentage of the community citizens will give strong support to the proposed family life and sex education program. It is necessary to point out that almost all communities have a small, vocal minority of people who will offer initial opposition to the program. It is extremely important that a concerted effort be made to talk with the dissenters, either individually or in groups, in an effort to secure their support. Often, individuals who are opposed to the program are unaware of the aims and objectives of the program. Some school districts have successfully appointed interested persons to speak to individuals and groups in an effort to help resolve some of the questions associated with the program. Members of the original planning committee should be in an excellent position to help discuss the aims, objectives and aspirations of the family life and sex education program.

All communities have individuals who hold a liberal point of view insofar as sex education is concerned, as well as other citizens with very conservative attitudes. Local committees should be careful not to be unduly influenced by either group. It is much wiser to start with what will be accepted by a majority of citizens at the local level and continue from that point.

In the final analysis, curriculum development boils down to the point of developing a sound plan and materials that will be as nearly as possible acceptable to the local citizens, the school administration and the board of education. Competent people at the local community level are in the best position to help judge those materials that will be most suitable for use in their local schools and communities.

The curriculum committee should be able to complete its work in twelve to fifteen months. Several school districts have found it advantageous to have this committee work for six to eight weeks during the summer one year in advance of the planned initiation of the program. The committee can then continue its work during the regular school year. The following summer can be used for finalizing the materials and for making the necessary plans for implementing the program in the fall.[5]

The scope of the program will be determined by the curriculum committee, based on the information received by it from the parents and from the advisory committee. In subsequent chapters a basic curriculum is outlined, derived from various sources, that your curriculum committee may decide to utilize as a starting point, or which you may even decide to use in its present state. It will prove valuable, we are sure, as you develop your program.

Summary

In the organization of a sex education program, initial interest must be developed, sparked by either school personnel or members of the community. It is suggested that an informal exploratory committee be established to bring in a preliminary report. If this is well-received, a community planning committee

---

[5]*Steps Toward Implementing Family Life and Sex Education Programs in Illinois Schools.*

should be established to continue the exploratory work. If this is successful, a series of program objectives should be developed, and the program turned over to the curriculum committee for development of the actual curriculum. A sample curriculum that your committee should find useful is to be found in chapters 5 through 8.

CHAPTER 3

How to Implement the Sex Education Program

Many decisions must be made as the sex education program is developed. They will be discussed in this chapter.

Scheduling Family Life and Sex Education

Where should family life and sex education instruction be placed in the curriculum? This often perplexing and complicated problem must be resolved by the local district administration. A definite time allowance is mandatory if the instruction is to be meaningful and have continuity.

The elementary school presents minor problems in scheduling when compared with the junior and senior high school. In the elementary school, family life and sex education instruction should be the responsibility of the classroom teacher. Because of the flexibility that the self-contained classroom offers, it is not difficult to find time for instruction. Sex education may be taught as a unit of the health or science sequence, or it may be correlated with other appropriate subjects. When the correlation procedure is used, it is vitally important that plans be developed to insure that all teachers are adhering closely to the curriculum plan in order that repetition and omission will not occur. Many schools have found it advantageous to select one teacher to serve as a co-ordinator.

The junior high school level presents a multitude of problems in scheduling family life and sex education. Theoretically, there are many subject matter areas that have a legitimate relationship to and an interest in family life and sex education. It may be integrated with physical education, biology, home economics, social science, health education and very possibly other areas. There are many advantages to integrating instruction. The students will receive instruction from many different teachers and will be exposed to different points of view, and individual teachers will handle only those aspects of the topic in which they have specialization and competence. The disadvantage is that unless the most careful coordination is provided, there are apt to be gaps in instruction and endless repetition.

There is also an urgent need for a summing-up portion of time where all points of view can be carefully analyzed and, hopefully, desirable attitudes developed. In those schools that offer a one-semester health education course, the summing-up process should logically constitute a portion of the content of that course.[1]

Placing the Program in the Health Education Area

In the state of Delaware Department of Public Instruction's guide ("Health Education Curriculum Guide—A Comprehensive Program Kindergarten through Grade Twelve"), the Introduction to the guide and listing of objectives shows exactly how sex education, although not expressly called that, is integrated into the health education curriculum.

Introduction

The aim of health education is to prepare each pupil in Delaware to think logically and constructively about his present

---

[1] *Steps Toward Implementing Family Life and Sex Education Programs in Illinois Schools.*

and future health in order to stimulate him to develop positive patterns for decision making when coping with today's problems.

The schools have a responsibility to assist each pupil to develop an understanding about himself and his environment to help him lead a more purposeful life.

A comprehensive program of health education in grades K-12 establishes a framework for meeting the health needs, the interests and problems of pupils, as well as preparing them for their role as future parents and dynamic citizens.

Health as a unified concept must be approached with consideration for the total human being and the variety of forces that affect health behavior. Health is concerned with attitudes, knowledge and practices of the individual, his family and community.

The health education program is based on the three processes—growing and developing, interacting, and decision making—that are typical of every individual regardless of age, sex, occupation or social status.

Growing and developing is a "dynamic life process by which the individual is in some ways like all other individuals, in some ways like some other individuals, and some ways like no other individual."

Interacting is "an ongoing process in which the individual is affected by and in turn affects certain biological, social, psychological, economic, cultural and physical forces in the environment."

Decision making is "a process unique to man of consciously deciding to take or not to take an action, or choosing one alternative rather than another."[2]

Objectives

1. To prepare the individual to learn to cope effectively with his problems in present-day society.
2. To assist the individual to develop desirable attitudes and practices along with an appreciation of health principles.
3. To stimulate critical thinking on moderation and self-control in one's daily behavior.

---

[2]School Health Education Study.

4. To help the individual to realize that everyone has different levels of abilities and needs as well as problems of adjustment to make.
5. To assist the individual to accept the strengths and weaknesses of his peers.
6. To prepare the individual to think critically on recommendations made for health products and health services.[3]

Alaska, Michigan and Minnesota, as well as many other states, place sex education in the health education area.

Placing the Program in the Subject Areas

In the New York City curriculum, family living and sex education is not a discrete curriculum area but is taught in relation to such subject areas as language arts, science, social studies, home economics and health education. Classroom living and daily situations involving interpersonal relationships apart from any particular subject area frequently offer the teachable moment to develop a given generalization most naturally and effectively. For these reasons the teacher is the best judge of how much time to give to the implementation of any generalization, providing the curriculum adequately stresses the importance of doing so.

Grade Placement

The allocation of the generalizations to a grade block rather than to a specific grade enables the teacher to select for instructional purposes those generalizations that are appropriate for the children in his class and relevant to their needs and interests. This is particularly true for teachers of prekindergarten and kindergarten children. Teachers will find that some of the material not presented to the entire group may be of use in answering individual questions. The maturity levels of pupils and the socio-

---

[3]Health Education Curriculum Guide, State of Delaware, prepared by Mrs. Edith Vincent, 1972.

cultural backgrounds of the families that form the school community are factors to be considered in the selection of content and suggested learning activities.

The following is a sample of a unit in science and health education. It is taken from the New York City curriculum guide.

Sample Science and Health Education Unit

Preadolescents are very much interested in and concerned about their physical growth and development. The rapid spurt in growth and the many changes accompanying it often result in anxieties concerning physical development. Young people at this age need information and guidance to help them accept their changing, maturing selves, and an opportunity to discuss freely their concerns about pubertal development.

This unit has been designed to satisfy these needs. A variety of visual aids and printed materials will help to provide factual information. Through the guidance of the teacher the anxieties of the students can be lessened and the development of wholesome attitudes effected. The unit should be developed for each class in terms of its particular needs and interests. Separate classes may be conducted for boys and girls where desirable.

Unit: *Physical Aspects of Puberty and Adolescence*

Content and Development		
Objectives	Evaluation	Grades: 5, 6
Approach	Sample Lesson Plan	
Development	Instructional Materials	Time: 3-4 weeks
Activities		

Objectives

1. To develop an acceptance of one's emerging human sexuality. This includes the physical and emotional changes of puberty, plus the significance of sex in our society.

2. To acquire knowledge of the physical aspects of pubertal growth and development.
3. To understand that the changes that occur during adolescence prepare boys and girls for their roles as men and women.
4. To become aware of the uniqueness of individual growth patterns.
5. To realize that all human beings go through the same stages in their life cycle.
6. To understand the interrelationships of physical, social and emotional growth patterns.

Approach

Show pictures of typical adolescents and of seven- or eight-year-old children. Elicit from pupils the observable likenesses and differences between the two groups, and note the fact that the differences in appearance are related to differences in age. Ask the pupils what they think causes the changes as one grows from childhood into adolescence. Why are these changes so important?

Ask: What is a typical fifth [sixth] grader like? Give the pupils the opportunity to talk about their ideas. List the characteristics that are discussed.

Ask: How are fifth [sixth] graders different from those in the third grade? What changes have taken place? What causes these changes? What will these fifth [sixth] graders be like when they are in the seventh [eighth] grade?

Show pictures of baby boys, baby girls, men and women. Ask: How do these babies become men and women? What does growing up mean?

Encourage the pupils to discuss the various ways in which a person matures.

Ask: How does your body change as you grow up?

Development

1. The rate of growth for each individual varies during his lifetime.

2. The most rapid periods of growth after birth are during the first year and during preadolescence.
3. Many changes occur during the preadolescent period.
4. The age at which puberty begins varies with individuals.
5. The major changes that take place at puberty are caused by the hormones from the pituitary glands and the sex glands (testes and ovaries).
6. Girls usually reach puberty at an earlier age than boys.
7. The female reproductive system includes a pair of ovaries, two Fallopian tubes, a uterus and a vagina.
8. Although eggs are present in a girl's ovaries when she is born, the eggs do not begin to ripen until she reaches puberty. At that time, the menstrual cycle begins.
9. Many physical changes take place during the menstrual cycle.
10. There are many physical changes at puberty, including the development of the secondary sexual characteristics.
11. In boys, the testes begin to produce sperm at puberty. Nocturnal emissions may begin at this time.

Activities

Using pictures of preadolescents, show variations in body build. Discuss reasons for differences.

Have a buzz session: What is a typical teenager like?

Make lists of changes that take place in boys and in girls at puberty.

Ask the pupils to bring in pictures of themselves at an earlier age. Discuss the physical changes that have taken place.

After teacher sets up a question box, have pupils submit questions they would like to have answered by the teacher.

Find out how the glands affect pubertal development. Use charts or transparencies to show location of the glands.

Use charts or transparencies to review the menstrual cycle.

Make a graph of the heights of boys and girls. Discuss reasons for differences among the boys, among the girls, between boys and girls.

Discuss the reasons that some boys and girls reach puberty later than others in their age group.

Talk about the ways in which pubertal changes can affect social
life.

Write a description of a typical teenager.

What health rules should teenagers follow?

Make a list of recreational activities for teenagers.

Use filmstrips, charts, and/or transparencies of the male reproductive system to show the changes that occur at puberty.

Compare male and female pubertal development.

Discuss: Why is the period of adolescence often called the
"years of change"?

Bring in advertisements of products recommended for teenagers. Discuss the use and merit of these products.

Discuss why teenagers especially need good diets and sufficient
rest.

Visit the Hall of Man, American Museum of Natural History, to
see materials on the reproductive systems and growth
patterns in males and females.

Evaluation

Have each member of the class write a brief composition
comparing himself to the average teenager.

Have pupils prepare a checklist of physical changes occurring
during puberty.

Give a knowledge test of the biological terms related to
puberty.

Sample Lesson Plan

Topic: The Female Reproductive System—Menstruation*

Objectives

To learn that the menstrual cycle begins at puberty.

To understand that menstruation is one sign that a girl is
becoming a woman and that she may be able to have
children.

---

*Separate classes for boys and girls, where desirable. The same content, however,
should be taught to both groups.

To be aware of the fact that each girl develops into womanhood at her own rate.

To learn about the physical changes that take place during the menstrual cycle.

To realize that menstruation is a normal and natural function.

Materials

1. Charts or series of pictures of females in various stages of the life cycle.
2. Chart or transparency of the female reproductive system.
3. Film or filmstrip on menstruation.

Motivation

Use a chart or series of pictures showing stages in a female's life cycle.

Teacher: During a lifetime all of us go through various stages. The first stage after birth is this (show picture of baby or refer to chart).

Ask: "What will the next stage be?" Elicit from children what the next two stages will be. "This is the stage at which you are now [preadolescence]. How is a person at this stage different from a toddler? This is the stage you will soon be at [adolescence]. What are some of the signs that you are reaching this stage?"

Development

Show film or filmstrip on menstruation. "Let's look at the film [filmstrip] that will help you understand some of the changes occurring at this time in a girl's life."

Ask: What is puberty? At what age does puberty begin?

How does a girl know when she has reached puberty?
What parts of the body are involved in the process of menstruation?

Use a chart or transparency of the female reproductive system. Ask the pupils to point out the ovaries, the Fallopian tubes, the uterus and the vagina.

Ask: What is in the ovaries? When do these eggs begin to ripen? How many eggs usually ripen at one time? [Introduce the word "ovulation."] How often do the eggs ripen? What happens after an egg leaves the ovary?

Have students trace the path of the egg after it breaks out of its follicle in the ovary.

Ask: What happens in the uterus when the egg leaves the ovary? Why is there a thickening of the lining of the uterus? What happens if the egg is fertilized?

Use a filmstrip, transparency or chart to show the thickened uterine lining, the path of the egg to the uterus and the embedding of the egg in the lining.

Ask: What happens if the egg is not fertilized?

Use a filmstrip, transparency or chart to indicate the path of the egg, its disintegration and the menstrual flow.

Ask: How long does the menstrual flow last?

[Point out that the menstrual period refers to the length of the menstrual flow.]

Give the pupils an opportunity to ask questions and to discuss them.

Summary

1. What is meant by menstruation?
2. Why is the beginning of menstruation a sign that a girl can become a mother?
3. How should a girl take care of herself when she is menstruating? (This question might lead to a separate lesson on this topic.)

Conclusion

This is the time in your life when you are growing up, when there are many changes in your body. However, it is important for you to understand how and why you are changing. Although you've learned some of the ways that you change from girlhood to womanhood, there may still be questions you want answered. Write them down, and we will answer them in our next lesson. If you think of any other questions later on, hand them in, too. Don't put your name on the paper.

Note: The same information should be planned for boys' classes.

Note: A follow-up unit might be: How do the physical changes that occur at puberty and during adolescence affect an individual's emotional and social development?

Books

For Pupils

Beck, L. *Human Growth.* N.Y.: Harcourt, Brace & World, 1959.
DeSchweintz, Karl. *Growing Up.* N.Y.: Macmillan, 1965.
Gruenberg, S. *The Wonderful Story of You.* N.Y.: Doubleday, 1960.
Hofstein, S. *The Human Story.* N.Y.: Scott, Foresman, 1968.
Lerrigo, M., and H. Southard. *What's Happening to Me?* N.Y.: Dutton, 1956.[4]

The Incidental Approach

In many schools, and particularly in the lower grades, an incidental approach is used. The teachers answer any questions that the children may bring up. Lessons may be prepared or may be done spontaneously as the need for information arises. If this approach is used, we believe there should be some structuring of the classroom situation so that questions do arise, and so that the suggested material is covered. Since the sex education curriculum you develop within your school should be a continuing one, some specific topics must be covered. Even with an incidental approach it is necessary that the topics be, in some way, introduced into the curriculum.

---

[4]"Family Living Including Sex Education," Bureau of Curriculum Development, Board of Education, City of N.Y. 1969-1970 series. Used by permission.

Choosing the Staff

Especially relevant to the area of family living and sex education is the teacher's capacity to listen perceptively and to experience relative comfort in dealing with the conflicting, deeply rooted, emotional attitudes that are associated with family and sex. In this program more than in any other, the teacher's contribution of factual information is less significant than his or her skill in creating a climate that enables youngsters to deal constructively with issues that are intensely personal and relevant to their daily lives. His or her recognition of the possibilities of pupil growth and rapport with the class are the key to the success of this program.

It is difficult to be nonjudgmental and somewhat objective about sex. Yet, the teacher's nonjudgmental objectivity is a requirement for helping youngsters to sort out confusions and to develop slowly a set of internally integrated values that may be relied upon as bases for important decision making immediately and in the future.[5]

If one wishes a series of criteria to apply to teachers being considered for teaching sex education, these, we believe, would be of value:

1. Is the teacher able to develop rapport with members of both sexes? (A man's man might be fine with boys, but not with girls.)
2. Is this teacher interested in teaching this program, and motivated to do a good job with it? (If a person isn't, he or she will not prove adequate.)
3. Is the teacher willing to take the time and make the effort to educate himself or herself—to become as knowledgeable as possible?
4. Is the teacher interested in individuals as individuals? (Some teachers, for example, never even learn the names of all of the children in their classes. Some children, of course—the outgoing ones—but the quiet ones, never.)

---

[5] "Family Living Including Sex Education," City of New York, pp. 3, 4.

5. Does the teacher have the time to devote to creating a good program? (Some teachers are so involved with working toward their master's degrees, for example, that they haven't the time they need for the sex education program.)
6. Is the teacher a stable person? (Often people with many problems of their own seek to become counselors and even psychiatrists. If the teacher being considered is beset with personal problems such as a broken marriage, drinking or gambling, we feel he or she should be involved in teaching areas other than this.)
7. Can this teacher develop a give-and-take with the youngsters? Can he or she keep quiet some of the time, and listen to the youngsters? (We all know teachers who talk every minute! This would be disastrous in the sex education program.)
8. Is this teacher creative? Highly creative teachers can make this program very rewarding. It shouldn't be taught "from the textbook."

Providing Strong Administrative Leadership

In a program as controversial as sex education, there is a great need for a strong administrator. Since the superintendent has many, many things requiring his attention, it is suggested that he choose a coordinator. After this individual is selected, who should also be a strong person, the superintendent should make his feelings known to his coordinator who can then handle the flack. Rest assured there will be some! One of the tasks of the coordinator is to keep the superintendent informed of any and all developments. This can be done in writing, with a simple note as to how each matter was handled.

The coordinator is often the person selected to do the teacher selection and the teacher training.

Teacher Training

The most important role in implementing the sex education program, after the curriculum has been developed, is that played by the teacher. School districts can look to colleges and universities for assistance in training teachers to effectively teach family life and sex education.

Many teachers in contemplating teaching sex education feel that they are inadequate to handle the subject matter. However, reports from school districts throughout the nation indicate that most teachers with relatively short periods of training will gain confidence and competence in teaching family life and sex education. As a matter of fact, many will develop great skill. It has been found that many teachers who are reluctant in the beginning to teach sex education and family life find that they enjoy it after having gone through the material a time or two. In reviewing reports from throughout the nation, it would appear that on the average, one teacher in twelve will be unable to teach sex education for a variety of reasons. This does not pose a serious problem in the elementary school because teachers frequently trade assignments. Teachers with ability in music, but with less skill in physical education, have been successful in working out mutually acceptable exchanges for years.

After the curriculum has been constructed and the school district knows the materials that will be used, including visual aids and pamphlet material, it is most desirable that an in-service workshop be held for teachers. Many school districts have found that in a relatively short period of time, perhaps five two-hour sessions, teacher competence for teaching sex education can be improved. In-service training programs are also invaluable in giving teachers confidence for the task ahead. In-service workshops follow many different patterns. Regardless of how they are planned, they have many similarities.

The following list of topics are frequently included in the in-service training programs:

(1) A discussion of the need for family life and sex education in the school district.
(2) A discussion of mental health and emotional needs of school-age youth.
(3) A discussion of sex attitudes and behaviors in contemporary society.
(4) A discussion of the overall aims and objectives of the program and how the school district hopes to accomplish

these aims and objectives through an organized program of instruction.

(5) A discussion of the basic biological, psychological and sociological aspects of sexuality.

(6) A discussion of values and standards as they relate to school-age youth.

(7) A discussion and preview of all the instructional materials to be used in the program.

(8) A discussion of concerns of teachers and of anticipated teacher problems.

(9) A discussion by a teacher who has taught in a successful family life and sex education program.

Almost all schools have discovered that after the unit on sex education and family life has been taught one time, it is desirable for the teachers to evaluate the material. Quite often schools revise the curriculum after the material has been taught once, deleting those experiences that did not work well and expanding successful experiences. Also, difficult questions asked by students can be accumulated and expert advice secured in finding answers to these questions. Teachers are consistent in pointing out that groups of students tend to ask many of the same questions over and over again.

School districts should be able to find resource people to help with the in-service program in local communities. In many cases, a local physician interested in the program will be happy to discuss the basic biological facts. This could, however, be done by a person from the science department. Priests, ministers and rabbis are generally willing to discuss their views insofar as values, attitudes and behavioral standards are concerned. Universities and colleges have competent psychologists, sociologists and health educators on their staffs whose services can be secured.

There are people with competence in mental health in a variety of state agencies. These people are usually willing to lend assistance. It is helpful if a teacher can be found who has taught in a successful family life and sex education program. One presentation from such a person will do much to dispel the fears and anxieties that are common among teachers.

School districts should approach the in-service workshop with the idea that all are going to learn together. Periodic evaluations by districts with ongoing programs have indicated that teachers considered the in-service training to be the most helpful aspect of the entire developmental process in gaining teacher support for the program.[6]

The New York City teacher training course is described as follows.

In-service courses should present a variety of approaches and techniques, enriched subject matter, and a diversified range of teaching materials.

The courses should include: pooling of ideas and experiences, evaluation of lesson plans and lessons, and examination of curriculum materials in family life and sex education; the use of specialists (physicians, psychologists, social workers, family life educators, etc.), panel discussions, supplementary literature, field trips to community resources (daycare centers, museums, zoos, etc.), and audio-visual materials. Current materials should be introduced on a continuing basis for the purposes of viewing, evaluating and adapting.

Special Training for Teachers

The emphasis on attitudes as part of the process as well as the goal of this program suggests that special approaches to teacher preparation may be useful. Laboratory training techniques including opportunities to experience interpersonal relationships and group processes are examples of appropriate special preparation.

Laboratory training experiences are designed to help normal individuals learn more about themselves and other people. These include verbal and nonverbal experiences, conceptualizations, theoretical formulations concerning issues and process, and ex-

----

[6]*Steps Toward Implementing Family Life and Sex Education Programs in Illinois Schools*, pp. 20, 21.

periences within unstructured small groups. Through such experiences, attention is directed to a variety of personal and social-interaction issues. Activities might include practice in assuming another's point of view, in giving and receiving help, or in managing conflict. Laboratory training methods develop conditions that permit such interactions to be experienced and to be examined. The participants are then enabled to experiment with various role models for coping more effectively in these areas.

The small groups deal with the here and now in the group life of the participants. The members develop a shared responsibility and interest that forms the milieu within which they learn to be direct and honest in dealing with their own reactions. This supports their practice in trying out new behaviors. As the group deals with itself in this way, individuals become more attuned to their own feelings, attitudes and reaction patterns. They are also able to study the impact they have on others, and to learn how they can be more effective in dealing with others. They become aware of the many levels of meaning communicated by themselves and by those with whom they interact. As the participants grow in awareness, they grow in acceptance of self and acceptance of others.

Laboratory training experiences are facilitated by a psychologist, a social worker or a psychiatrist who has acquired special skills. He helps the participants create optimal conditions for emotionally anchored learning. He helps members of the group identify significant interactions and to generalize from their own experiences in the group. One of his most significant contributions is the help given to the group in how to use themselves and their co-members as sources of learning. This is an alternative to reliance on the traditional authority represented by a group leader.

The teacher who has experienced laboratory training can apply his understanding of the differences between influence and control, between candor and self-deception, between trust and wariness, between strengthening acceptance and weakening attack. He is equipped to guide his pupils to use their own and each other's resources. He can help his students integrate factual information and work their way through conflict and confusion to enlightenment. He is more likely to develop the kind of classroom climate in which such goals of the program may be achieved.

The content of the program touches many sensitive pressure points for teacher and pupil. Family relationships and matters pertaining to sex cannot be and should not be so objectified that this is not the case. The laboratory method of participation in interpersonally directed learning experiences is a special type of training for handling a special program. The coordinators and guidance personnel charged with the development and initial supervision of the program have been participants in such training sessions. Efforts should be made to provide similar experiences for all teachers who will implement this curriculum.[7]

As you can see, there is great variation here. Certainly both techniques may be utilized.

Continuing In-service Education

As with every successful program, an ongoing program of in-service education is a necessity. One of the main reasons for this is the sharing of information among teachers. Lessons that look excellent on paper may turn out to be duds, whereas others that do not look so promising catch the youngsters' imaginations and prove to be very effective. It is worthwhile to ask your teachers to keep track of their results in this regard, particularly noting those lessons that can be given to other teachers for other classes, and those that should be redeveloped.

Another reason for the ongoing program is that new materials are constantly becoming available—kinescopes, for example. We must keep in mind that sex education and family living encompass a large area of man's interest, and programs of the development of living things other than human (and human, of course) can add greatly to the program.

Teachers should be encouraged to discuss their own particular problems in regard to their teaching, and a place to ventilate them can be tremendously important. The degree of embarrassment teachers feel at first diminishes for most, but not for all of

---

[7]"Family Living Including Sex Education," City of New York, pp. 3, 4.

them. For the latter, a course and a place to work out some of this emotion can prove very valuable.

The sharing of pupil- or teacher-made materials is another function of in-service workshops. It is hardly necessary for every teacher to invent the wheel. As a teacher comes up with worthwhile material, it can be passed around to others teaching the subject.

Continuing education also presents the opportunity to hear many speakers—experts in allied fields who can help by increasing the teachers' knowledge and approach to this knowledge. The more your teachers know about this, or any subject, the better a job they will do when teaching it. Sex education is an area where people are reluctant to admit they need information, and, therefore, by placing it before them, much can be accomplished.

Selecting Materials

The state of Michigan offers the following guidelines.

---

1. An effective program makes appropriate use of the many resources available on the local, state and national levels. However valuable a resource may be in many areas, it should be viewed in the context of its value for a specific purpose. Resources should be selected in terms of their appropriateness to specific purposes.

2. Technical resource personnel should be used to assist the teacher, help in evaluation of materials, help interpret programs to the parents, provide counseling for students, help in in-service education activities, and serve as members of the School-Community Sex Education Committee and/or curriculum committee.

3. The educational value of each resource should be assessed in addition to factors of cost, accessibility and the time involved in its use.

4. It is desirable to formulate policies and guidelines concerning the effective and appropriate use of these resources. This can be accomplished by developing a resource guide listing sources of potential assistance with suggestions on their most profitable use.

5. Inasmuch as resource materials vary a great deal in quality and cost and may not in instances be suitable for public school use, a sound plan for the systematic review and evaluation of materials in terms of teaching objectives is wise.

6. It would be desirable to develop a comprehensive library of curriculum resources for teacher use in self-improvement, program development and implementation. Materials in the library should be provided especially for parents' use.

7. In view of the variety of grades and the number of students likely to be involved in a program of sex education, it is important to have sufficient materials available. However, appropriate restrictions and controls should govern the use of these materials.

8. Potential problems associated with the use of materials by students indicate that the development and use of such a collection of materials should be carefully considered from all viewpoints.

9. It would be desirable to make short- and long-range plans to budget for the sex education materials needed to help realize the objectives of the program.

10. Once the curriculum framework and resources for the program have been developed, recommendations concerning the need for specific materials would be justified and, depending upon available funds, priorities could be established for their purchase and/or rental.

11. School personnel in charge of curriculum should take the necessary steps to secure proper facilities and equipment for operating the materials resource program. This would help insure maximum efficiency in the use of learning activities and learning resources.[8]

Once the curriculum committee has developed a program, it must, we believe, be approved by the board of education.

Every school district that anticipates inaugurating a program in sex education should have the firm, *written* approval of the local board of education. It is impossible to overemphasize this

[8]"Sex Education and Family Information," State of Michigan Department of Education, Lansing, 1971. Used by permission.

point. Strong approval and support by the board of education gives status to sex education and family life instruction. It is also reassuring to the teachers and to the administration that in the event problems arise, they will have this high-level backing. Schools that are attempting to offer instruction in family life and sex education without the written approval of the board of education are in a very insecure position. Problems will arise from time to time that may need to be considered by the board.

A problem all districts must resolve is that centered around provisions for exempting certain students from sex education instruction on the basis of constitutional or other grounds. Local boards of education and the school administration should consider this matter very carefully and establish written policies regarding exemption, if any. There will undoubtedly be some variation from one school district to another on this point.

Most of the difficulties that arise in the area of family life and sex education will be those associated with students mis-understanding or misinterpreting information that the teacher has given. There is apt to be an occasional error in judgment by a teacher. All too often, students will not go to the teacher for clarification but will report to the parents or perhaps the school administration. The parents frequently go directly to the board of education with a complaint. Obviously, the board of education must have been informed of and have approved the entire program that has been planned.[9]

Community and Parental Approval

As has already been stated, the need for community approval is one that no district planning a sex education program can ignore. *It is critical to the success of the program.* In the case of the Parsippany-Troy Hills Township Schools (New Jersey), the statements of approval are included in their book, "Human Sexuality: An Instructional Guide."

One decision that must be made is to decide whether or not every child must be given sex education if it is approved by the

---

[9]*Steps Toward Implementing Family Life and Sex Education Programs in Illinois Schools*, pp. 18, 19.

parents as a group. The alternative is to offer alternate instruction. This matter is one of extreme importance and must be decided upon before the program can be instituted.

***

Initiating the Program

There should be little difficulty associated with initiating the program in family life and sex education if the proper developmental procedures have been followed. Above all, the school district should not attempt to glamorize sex education instruction but should approach it as any other subject matter area.

The emotional climate in which instruction is to take place is important. The teacher, of course, has the primary responsibility for developing an appropriate atmosphere. It is a good idea to delay sex education instruction until the teacher has had an opportunity to establish rapport with the class as a group and with its members individually. This is important at all grade levels.

The most difficult aspect of teaching family life and sex education is centered around student questions. Class discussion is important and should be encouraged. However, students may, on occasion, ask questions or raise topics that are inappropriate for general class discussion. Teachers should not be reluctant to refer students to appropriate sources, sometimes outside the school, for answers.

Teachers will frequently be asked questions that they cannot answer simply because they do not know the answers. In such cases, the better part of valor is for the teacher to frankly admit he or she doesn't know, but can always find the answer at a later time. The giving of misinformation is devastating and if done to excess can jeopardize the program.

It is important that all school personnel be well-informed about the program, including those who are not actually teaching it. All school personnel should give the same loyal support to this program as to other school programs.[10]

***

[10]*Steps Toward Implementing Family Life and Sex Education Programs in Illinois Schools*, pp. 21, 22.

It is a known fact that the most difficult problem associated with developing programs in family life and sex education is getting started. It is hoped that this book will assist interested school districts in organizing and planning programs that will have strong community support and that will make a substantial contribution to the total education of their youth.

Summary

Among the decisions that must be made in regard to the sex education program as it is being developed is its placement in the curriculum. In the elementary schools this does not present a serious problem, but in the junior high school grades it does. Many school districts have placed it in the health education area. Others have not placed it in any particular area; it is covered in the subject area taught by the teacher trained for it.

The choice of the staff for teaching the sex education program is of particular importance, with certain personality traits essential. Probably of prime import is the ability of the teacher to develop rapport with both boys and girls. Creativity and respect for each individual child are vital, as well, if the program is to succeed. The training of the teachers is one of the points that must be focused upon in both factual material and in attitudes. It is suggested that continuing in-service workshops or courses be offered to teachers in the sex education program. A listing of guidelines for the selection of resource materials is included. Once the program has been developed by the curriculum committee, written approval of the local school board is a necessity before the program is initiated. Then, as the sex education program becomes operative, a constant process of evaluation should occur. This is described in chapter 10.

CHAPTER 4   *How to Communicate the Sex Education Program to Parents*

As has been stated previously, parental cooperation in the sex education program is a must. No program of so personal a nature can possibly exist without true parental involvement. It is important to include parent representatives in all phases of the planning of the sex education program in order to explore their feelings about the needs of their children.

Once a sex education curriculum has been decided upon and accepted by the school board, the next decision to be made is whether or not every child is to be included in the program. If the answer is yes, then permission forms are unnecessary. If the answer is no, then a form should be sent out, or, better still, parents should be invited to a meeting. At this meeting the sex education program should be described once again in detail and the permission forms distributed.

When parents refuse to allow their children to participate, it may be because of deep personal conviction, or because they are unaware of the actual course—what their children will be learning or how the topics will be handled. In the case of the former, we believe their wishes should be respected. In the case of the latter, we suggest the use of materials such as that which follows.

Notifying Parents About the Particular
Curriculum Being Used

The Belleville Public Schools, District #118 sent out a brochure to every parent of a first grader. It is extremely specific and leaves no doubt whatsoever as to the content the teacher will cover. There are similar brochures for every grade.

BELLEVILLE PUBLIC SCHOOLS
DISTRICT #118
BELLEVILLE, ILLINOIS

November 6, 1976

Dear Parents:

The Health Program in District #118 attempts to provide instruction to the student in all phases of his growth and development, whether it be physical, social or emotional growth. This instruction is geared to the needs of children at their own age level. Part of the health program includes a short unit in family living and sex education.

In order to maintain good communication with the home, you will find attached a packet containing the introduction, philosophy, and a listing of objectives, activities and materials that will be used *by the teacher* in the implementation of the family living program at your child's grade level. Also included is a permission slip, which should be signed and returned to your child's teacher by November 17.

The instructional unit will begin on February 5th and possibly extend through February 16th. It should be noted that this year's program is a repeat of last year's. No changes have been made.

If you have questions, please discuss them with your child's teacher.

INTRODUCTION

The Health Committee of the Belleville Public Schools District #118 has developed a proposed curriculum in "Family Living and Sex Education" to supplement our new Scott, Foresman health textbooks. This program was approved by the Board of Education at its regular monthly meeting on May 18, 1976.

It is felt that the concepts, when implemented, will help boys and girls establish more positive attitudes toward themselves, their growing bodies, and their peer and family groups. We hope they will be able to make responsible decisions about their sexual nature as they grow up to assume appropriate places in their adult society. It is our aim to give vocational guidance for family living.

A child who completes the kindergarten through eighth year sequence should have a good understanding of the biology of human reproduction, the area indicated by parents as the most difficult one for them to discuss with their children.

The curriculum relies on repetition to reinforce the material presented at previous grade levels. We believe the repetition is essential because of the wide range of interest and maturity within each classroom. Each time the material is repeated, it is presented with different supplemental materials appropriate for the grade level.

We feel the Curriculum Committee for this project should be a continuing one. Revisions and/or additions should improve the program when possible. Supplemental materials must be excellent in content and presentation. Appropriate materials must be available to the teachers.

We present this draft of Instructional Guidelines for Family Living with the stipulation that satisfactory in-service training for the teachers before the program can begin.

FAMILY LIVING PHILOSOPHY

We believe that "Family Living" is an important part of the total curriculum in District #118. The content of the subject is readily integrated in social studies and health education, including growth and development and the reproductive system.

The instruction in Family Living is designed to include more than understanding physical, mental, emotional, social, economic and psychological phases of human relations. It includes more than the necessary anatomical and reproductive information. The emphasis is on attitudes, development and guidance related to value judgments.

The family unit remains the unit of structure of our society. If good home life is to prevail, our hope lies in guiding people to experience the satisfaction of relating well to their mother, father, brothers and sisters. Children can be quite helpful in making the home a happy one. Respect for humankind begins early.

We believe that the creation of wholesome attitudes is far more important than remembering all the facts. Wholesome attitudes are the foundation of a strong moral character. Facts may be forgotten but emotional responses and attitudes that accompany the learning remain.

Education focused on fact giving is the approach when the problem is ignorance. Our goal is to impart appropriate information while helping pupils develop values on which to make their own decisions when exposed to choices that affect their health and total living experiences.

First Grade—Family Living Objectives

1. Accepts his responsibility as an important member of the family and a special helper.
2. Appreciates efforts of mother and father for family members and discusses different home patterns.
3. Develops sense of responsibility for own body.
4. Understands egg cell is basic to new life.
5. Learns that some animals hatch from eggs and others develop inside body of mother until birth.
6. Appreciates wonder of human body.

First Grade—Family Living Activities

For Objective No. 1:

1. See *Health and Growth,* Book I, T42-44.
2. Check home for safety—fire hazards, etc.
3. Make seasonal decorations for home.

For Objective No. 2:

1. Draw pictures of members of family and introduce family to

class through the picture (fun to do around Thanksgiving—draw family as pilgrims).

2. See *Health and Growth,* Book I, T42-44 (Unit 7).

For Objective No. 3:

1. Habits of cleanliness.
2. Dental care—a class-dictated story of the "Happy Tooth" giving rules for good dental care.
3. Make tissue faces along with talking about taking care of colds—see *Health and Growth,* T28-42.
4. Kellogg's breakfast contest.

For Objective No. 4:

1. Use microscope to see cells and examine simple plant life.
2. Combine discussion of amoeba with an art lesson on shapes.

For Objective No. 5:

1. Field trip to the Children's Zoo at Forest Park, if possible.
2. Fit the animals hatched from eggs into egg "frames" or "cracked eggs."
3. Use pictureforms to discuss which farm animals hatched or were born live.
4. Use National Dairy Council Study Print, "We All Like Milk," to learn about many animals who nurse their young.

For Objective No. 6:

1. Make a see-through man. Outline a life-sized child, using someone in the class as a model, on large mural paper. Then see how many organs the children can draw in and label.
2. Follow through with ditto—My Dictionary (page 50) can be used to help with labeling.
3. Rhyme for body parts (see below).

First Grade—Family Living

Find the body parts that rhyme with:
      1. phones   (bones)

First Grade—Family Living (continued)

2. tongue   (lung)
3. dart   (heart)
4. train   (brain)
5. hands   (glands)
6. river   (liver)
7. nine   (spine)
8. bibs   (ribs)

First Grade—Supplementary Materials

1. *Health and Growth,* Book I   Scott, Foresman Teacher's Manual

2. We All Like Milk   Ten Study Prints and Teacher's Guidebook— available upon request: National Dairy Council 2710 Hampton Avenue St. Louis, Missouri See nurse for order blanks.

3. *My Dictionary* (page 50)   Scott, Foresman & Company[1]

The same letter to the parent, introduction and family living philosophy accompany each grade level. Here is the information for grade 6.

Sixth Grade—Family Living Objectives

1. Understands cellular structures and their functional relationships (muscle, bone, nerve, skin, blood, reproductive).
2. Discusses anatomical and physiological differences among human beings.

---

[1]Belleville Public Schools, District #118, Belleville, Illinois. Used by permission.

3. Recognizes physiological and anatomical terminology.
4. Understands that emotions relate to biological functions.
5. Learns that boys and girls share the responsibility of emotional control and respect for each other.

Sixth Grade—Concepts for Study

  I. Human Physiology
 II. Glands Affecting Growth
III. Changes in Growth Due to Glands
IV. How Life Starts
 V. Heredity
VI. Family Structure

Sixth Grade—Family Living Activities

I   Human Physiology

  A. Cells
  B. Tissues
  C. Organs
  D. Body Systems

Activity: Chapter 7 in the health text should be studied prior to chapter 10. Good lead-up material.

Activity: Use microscope in the study of cells, blood, etc.

Activity: Correlate human physiology with art work and bulletin board displays.

Suggestion: Show filmstrip "Maturing Boys and Girls."

II.   Glands Affecting Your Growth

  A. Pituitary
  B. Reproduction glands

III.   Changes in Growth Due to Glands

  A. Physical
  B. Emotional

Activity: Write key phrases from the filmstrip "Maturing Boys and Girls" on the board and ask the class to respond to them with the first thing that comes to mind. (See Study Guide and Script.)

Activity: Large group, panel or buzz discussions on:

    a. What it means to grow up.
    b. Problems in relation to emotions.
    c. How to develop emotional control.
    d. Personal health practices corresponding to the physical changes.
    e. The implications of the admonition to boys that "boys don't cry" and "men don't cry."
    f. Ways of showing love and respect for friends, for members of family.
    g. Masculine and feminine roles in life.

Activity: Role playing

    a. Emotions and emotional control.
    b. Showing how one grows in responsibility.

Activity: Suggested essay topics:

    a. "Qualities I Like in Other Boys and Girls My Age"
    b. "The Personality of My Best Friend"
    c. "What Does It Mean to Be Popular?"
    d. "What Does It Mean to Be a Good Sport?"

Activity: Teacher reads to class articles dealing with fear, jealousy, anger, hurt feelings, etc.

Activity: Problem box—Students deposit brief descriptions of problems they have in getting along with members of their own age group or with members of their families. Class discussion or role playing of situations to help students improve their interpersonal relationships.

IV. How Life Starts

    A. Egg cell—ovum
    B. Sperm cell from father

C. Fertilization of egg

D. Embryonic and fetal developments

Suggestion: Introduce this topic with chapter 10 of the textbook.

V.   Heredity

A. Chromosomes—23 pairs

B. Genes—Determine color of hair, eyes, etc.

Suggestions: 1. Material covered in chapter 10 of text.
2. Small group research (human and animal gene characteristics).

VI.   Family Structure

A.   Importance of a family

B.   Mother-father role

1. Before parenthood
2. When parenthood begins

C.   Your place in the family

Sixth Grade—Supplementary Materials

1. "Maturing Boys and Girls" (filmstrip and guide)	Available in building. Appropriate for boys and girls to view together.
2. "It's Wonderful Being a Girl"	*For girls only.* Films available in Health Office.
3. "A Story About You" (pamphlet for pupils)	American Medical Association. One per teacher available, plus four copies for each sixth grade.
4. "Growing Up and Liking It" (booklet for girls)	Education Dept., Box A-68 Personal Products Company

Sixth Grade—Supplementary Materials (Continued)

Milltown, New Jersey 08850
(free)

5. *The Wonderful Story of*   Sidonie M. Gruenberg
   How You Were Born*   Hanover House
                        Garden City, New York[2]

A consent form you might wish to use, which would accompany the type of material described above, is as follows:

Dear _____ (fill in principal's name)

I hereby give permission for my child _____
_____ of class _____
to take part in the sex education and family living course now being offered at _____
School.

                 Sincerely yours,

              _____

              Parent signature
              (or guardian)

_____

Date

If there is some material to be used by individual students, as you may have noted in the section above, postscripts giving permission for each item separately should be listed.

---

[2]Belleville Public Schools, District #118, Belleville, Illinois.

*Teacher to keep in desk as a resource book. Some parents want their children to read the book. *If consent form is signed yes,* permit the capable and mature pupils to read the book.

Parent Workshops

One of the observations many professionals have made is they are shocked by the number of parents who need adult education in sex education and family living. Many adults have never had courses in these subjects, and have, indeed, gotten much of their information helter-skelter. Warren Gadpaille, M.D., writing in *The Family Coordinator* states: "When teaching classes in adult sex education programs, the author routinely finds parents to be woefully misinformed about the simplest details of sexual function. Adults still ask questions about the dire consequences of masturbation and are often very skeptical of reassurance."[3]

There is a tremendous need for comfortable, meaningful parental workshops where no one feels threatened. Children are receiving sex education from their earliest days. If a parent is guilt-ridden or troubled, this will certainly be transmitted to his or her child. Attitudes are learned by seeing examples. The way parents behave toward each other teaches the children far, far more than words. If parents are willing and able to discuss sexual matters comfortably with their children, then the subject takes on a wholesome aspect. If their parents are embarrassed, the children will be also.

In workshops, more than information about sex education should be conveyed. Attitudes toward family living must be worked on constantly. To put it concisely, workshops should help parents to see and therefore be able to transmit to their children the concept that normal and natural sexuality is acceptable in their eyes.

The parents must know exactly what the school program consists of so that they are not made to feel foolish if their children ask questions. Parents should be made aware of the materials being used—the textbooks, the charts, filmstrips, films and cassettes. You don't want your parents incredulously saying, "I never heard of such a thing," when a young boy or girl says, "We saw a film about menstruation today."

Your teachers need special, detailed instruction for teaching the youngsters *and* for teaching the parents as well. Teachers need

[3]Gadpaille, Warren J. "Parent-School Cooperation in Sex Education—How Can the Professional Help?" *The Family Coordinator*, Oct. 1970.

to know psychosexual development, sexual physiology and anatomy, information about homosexuality, and they should be
especially able to correct information about the myths and old
wives' tales. Women today are still slapping their daughter's faces,
as they did years ago, when the girls began to menstruate. We must
teach them, if they haven't learned it elsewhere, that this is indeed
a superstition.

You may find your parents will be more comfortable in
all-male or all-female classes. Again, this goes back to their
background as children, of course. Some of the lessons, however,
may be covered in mixed classes. Of course, children should be
taught that certain aspects of their parents' lives are personal, and
as such are kept private. However, these aspects must not be
allowed to seem secretive or dirty, and should be talked about in
terms of married people.

Planning a parents' series of workshops will take as much
time and effort as planning the students' classes—and is every bit
as necessary.

Rap Sessions with Teachers or Counselors for
Parents Who Need Them

Rap sessions, or working in close rapport with a teacher or
counselor on an individual or group basis, may be as necessary for
a parent as for a child. In this situation, though, guidelines have to
be established.

1. If the parent wishes to discuss school-related matters in
   connection with the sex education program, this is certainly a
   school matter, and teacher or counselor should be available.
2. If the parent wishes to discuss personal or family matters,
   which are basically unrelated to the school situation, then the
   parent should be referred to an outside agency.

The teacher should rely on the counselor to make this
referral.

Many times in rap sessions matters come up that are far more
involved and require much more time than either a teacher or a
school counselor can devote to them. If this should be the case,
and a referral is made, be sure the parent does not see this as

personal rejection. Impress him or her with the idea that specially trained personnel can be of more assistance. Encourage him or her to come back to see the teacher or counselor, but emphasize that treatment is needed that the school simply cannot make available.

CHAPTER 5   *The Sex Education Curriculum for the Primary Grades*

Levels of Psychosexual Development

It is particularly important for the teacher working in the area of family living and sex education to understand as fully as possible the levels of physical, psychological and social development of the children he is teaching. Knowing their interests and concerns, their strengths and inadequacies, enables the teacher to select the generalizations in family living including sex education for which children are ready; helps him to develop these generalizations most effectively; and guides him in his choice of appropriate books and audio-visual aids.

The teacher is urged, therefore, to become familiar with the psychosexual levels described in the pages that follow. Since children grow and mature at their own rate, they may exhibit characteristics of levels before or beyond that of their age group. It is helpful, for this reason, for the teacher to be familiar with the characteristics of children younger and older than the children he is teaching. This will enable him to further individualize instruction in family living including sex education.

The Four- to Five-Year-Old

The four- to five-year-old child is extremely self-centered. At this age when he is starting school, he is much more concerned with his own identity than with the characteristics or needs of others. As he progresses through the prekindergarten and the kindergarten stages, he develops a constantly increasing awareness of others. He is becoming more perceptive of the special character-istics of mothers and fathers, boys and girls, parents and other adults. He begins to realize slowly that others, too, have needs and rights, and that he may have to wait to have his own needs satisfied. This gives rise to conflict within himself, and clashes occur with parents, siblings, friends and teachers. His rages against a sense of frustration when he cannot have his own way are momentary but very intense. It is this process of being frustrated at times and of not having every wish satisfied that leads him to a realization of others as separate persons. A major task of the child during this period of growth is the establishment of his own personal identity.

It is difficult to give up the possessive ways of infancy: the egotism, the selfishness, and the petty jealousies, and to begin to make an adjustment to the demands of the world outside the home. The previous and earlier goals of gratification and attain-ment of pleasure begin to be forfeited to the claims of the external world. Postponement of immediate fulfillment of every desire is to be learned.

As the child assimilates the admonition to relinquish his childish behavior, he begins to acquire within himself standards more acceptable to adults, and these in turn become the values he cherishes and later judges others by as well.

Basic value orientation is formed during this period, an orientation that will influence future learning and behavior. The feelings a child has about others and his perception of the feelings they have about him depend on his feelings about himself. How he values himself is related to the feeling he has about his own body. Early attitudes toward the body form the foundation for later personality development. Characteristic of this age range is the child's growing curiosity about himself, his body, and his familial relationships. It is the age of questions. The questions are not idle; they represent deep ponderings resulting from his growing aware-ness of these relationships. "Where did I come from?" "How did I begin?" are typical questions that indicate his growing concern with himself as an individual.

One of the more striking characteristics of the young child is his capability for vivid fantasy. He has not yet developed sufficiently in his orientation to the real world to be able to counteract his fears and anxieties about his deeper feelings. Therefore, he turns to the world of play to work out some of them. Play is the safety valve for his hidden wishes and discharge of tensions. Working out his own conflicts allows the child to temper his behavior in real life.

This is a period of richly imaginative activity, during which some of the most bizarre misconceptions can be formed concerning physical facts. It is for this reason that simple and accurate information about the body and its functions should be presented. The youngster is naturally curious about his body and is interested in differences between his body and those of other children and adults. His interests include the social and cultural aspects as well as the biological aspects of sexual role differentiation. It is during this period that the child develops consistent masculine or feminine orientation. The crucial problem of the period lies in the child's need for acceptance of his curiosity and reinforcement of his sexual identification.

The Six- to Eight-Year-Old

The child from six to eight years of age is developing more reality-oriented modes of behavior than those found in early childhood. He is learning as he moves into the larger environment of school and community that he no longer has a favored position; he is one among many. He becomes more amenable to the idea of postponing gratification and of doing what is expected of him. The powerful drives he experienced previously have diminished as a result of the demands of his parents. To a large degree, he is no longer at the mercy of his instincts nor so personally engrossed with his own conflicts.

Realistic education by his parents or other adults responsible for him has changed him from an egotistical, demanding infant to a much more reasonable young person ready to turn his energy outward. His relationship to his parents improves, and gradually he becomes more detached from them as he gains new friends and engages in more group activities.

This is not to say that he no longer needs his parents. But, he now has them within himself in the form of an inner voice known as conscience. In the previous stage of his development, the child was constantly at odds with his parents who tried to "civilize" him by controlling his unacceptable behavior and by educating him to conform to society's demands. By the time he is six years old, he has, to a large degree, accepted his parents' standards, and these are transformed into values he will use throughout his life.

In redirecting his energy away from his own personal concerns toward external things, the child of six to eight becomes increasingly more interested in intellectual concerns and group activities. New friends and new relationships engage his time and energy now. In addition, he begins to explore the challenging community around him.

In attempting to understand and cope with a world of expanded demands and possibilities, the six-year-old sometimes tends to go to extremes. He can be quite touchy and humorless about challenges to his sexual identification. Responses in social situations become more markedly masculine or feminine with each year, until by age eight, some boys and girls may reject any semblance of friendship outside their own sex.

Although great sensitivity to criticism is present throughout the entire period, the volatility and extreme reaction of the six-year-old give way to more stability and calm by age seven. At this age receptivity to factual discussion, even about bodily functions, increases. The eight-year-old is even more at ease in communicating with adults and is better able to express sexual curiosity. Discussions of sexuality can be very embarrassing to youngsters during these years unless conducted in a very matter-of-fact fashion. They feel more comfortable when the focus is on social rather than on biological terms.

Verbal aggression, including the use of obscenities, is frequently observed but is usually more reflective of confusion and inadequate communication skills than of deep hostility. Classroom activities can profitably focus on the formation of attitudes of dignity and respect for sexual and other bodily functions, thus helping the youngster to build a sense of personal competence and self-esteem.

Children of this age are beginning to understand concepts of love and friendship. However, the child's approach to such understanding is generally in terms of role prescription. Discussions of complex feelings can be difficult or embarrassing.[1]

OUTLINE–For Very Young Children

Unit I. "Routine Toilet Procedures"

A. Introduce scientific names of related body parts and bodily functions.
B. Help child develop acceptable bathroom habits.
C. Help child develop a wholesome attitude toward his body.

Unit II. "The Nature and Purpose of the Family"

A. To bring children into the world and care for them.
B. To shape personalities, develop values, habits, and attitudes toward life.
C. To provide love, companionship, security, and protection for its members.
D. To guide individual members to understand, respect, and accept themselves.
E. To provide necessary food, shelter, and physical (material) needs for all its members.
F. To provide opportunities for the acceptance of responsibility and learning of respect for others.
G. To provide moral and spiritual values.

OUTLINE–For Young Children

Unit I. "Where Babies Come From"

A. Both mother and father have roles in reproduction.

1. A baby is a result of love and affection.
2. A baby grows from the union of two cells, one from the mother and one from the father.

---

[1] "Family Living Including Sex Education Guide," N.Y.C. Bureau of Curriculum Development, Board of Education, New York City, series 1969-1970. Used by permission.

B. Prenatal growth and birth is a miraculous process.

   1. A baby grows in a special place inside the mother's body called the uterus.

     a. It receives nourishment and oxygen through the umbilical cord.

     b. It receives protection within the pelvis and amniotic sac.

     c. It moves within the amniotic sac.

   2. A baby is born through a special opening called the birth canal.

     a. About nine months after the cells unite, the baby is ready to be born.

     b. Muscles help move the baby out.

     c. An average baby weighs about seven pounds and is about twenty inches long.

C. Human reproduction has deep meaning.

   1. Humans are knit together in a family unit.

   2. Human babies are loved and cared for.

   3. Humans are special and therefore have great responsibilities toward their families.

Unit II. "Growth and Development in Boys and Girls"

D. Boys and girls must have a concept of their role in society.

   1. Each must accept being the sex he is born.

   2. Each sex identifies his role with father or mother.

     a. Boys learn to be good fathers.

     b. Girls learn to be good mothers.

   3. Society often imposes different roles for girls and boys.

     a. Boys are often restricted from "feminine" activities.

     b. Girls are often restricted from "masculine" activities.

   4. Reason and circumstance should determine the role chosen.

E. Each person must discover and develop his self-concept.

   1. Each must discover his strengths and capabilities.

   2. Each must develop his interests and activities.

   3. Adults must encourage the attempts of children to understand their own feelings.

    4. Adults must encourage children to develop their own individuality.

F. Each person needs to be able to identify and understand the purpose of his external genitalia.

    1. The penis is the male external sex organ.
       a. It places sperm in the vagina.
       b. It passes urine from the body.
    2. The scrotum holds the testicles.
    3. The testicles produce sperm.
    4. The vulva is the region of the female external genitalia.
       a. It is an opening to let the sperm in.
       b. It is an opening to let the baby out.
       c. It assists in the passage of urine from the body.[2]

[2]*Guide for Teaching Health in the Area of Human Relations and Sexuality K-6, 8 and 11.* Independent School District No. 77, Mankato, Minnesota 56001, 1968. Used by permission.

The Curriculum

Grades 1 and 2

1. *Concepts:* The scientific names of body parts and related bodily functions should be used.

Learning Experiences: Attempt to discover the vocabulary that children already have for the body parts and bodily functions by informally noting requests for bathroom use. When children use incorrect terms, substitute the correct word in a quiet manner. Care should be taken not to ridicule or show shock at vulgar language. Give children an opportunity to pronounce the correct terms in a natural situation. Use correct terminology at every opportunity. Use the overhead transparency diagrams of related parts, with class discussion if questions come up in class. Tour the lavatory facilities in small groups on registration day. This may be a beginning point.

Audio-Visual Materials:

Slide: Statue by Verrocchio (p. 47 of *A Doctor Talks to Five to Eight Year Olds*).

2. *Concepts:* Handling of genitalia is natural and harmless.

Learning Experiences: When the circumstance of handling the genitals occurs, it should be treated in a warm, understanding manner, such as calmly redirecting the child's activity. It should not be treated in such a way as to cause the child to feel guilt. However, habitual sex play, when noted, requires the help and advice of qualified personnel.

Text and Library Books:

Starr, Helen M. and James Roger Fox. *Human Sexuality Education*. TAMA Division of Professional Productions, Inc. Suite 795, 608 2nd Ave. S., Minneapolis, Minnesota 55402.

3. *Concepts:* There are certain bathroom habits that are acceptable and necessary for good health.

Learning Experiences: Teacher and children develop ideas for bathroom procedures. These might include:

1. Using proper terms when requesting permission to go to the toilet.
2. Checking to see if someone is in toilet. Place extra chair at toilet door. Wait here if someone is in. If no one is in the chair, check on lavatory.
3. Using toilet properly.
   a. Close the door behind you.
   b. Keep toilet seat dry, clean, and neat. Boys lift seat when they urinate.
   c. Use toilet paper. Wipe anus from front to back after bowel movement.
   d. Flush toilet properly after use.
   e. Wash hands.
   f. Leave toilet room neat and clean.

The teacher may wish to handle this in a one-to-one informal relationship between teacher and child; or in a group discussion of how and why little girls sit in the bathroom, and conduct themselves, and why little boys stand. Mention could also be made of developing a habit of closing zippers before leaving the privacy of the bathroom. Later in the year discuss the use of upper grade lavatories (urinals, etc.). Use upper grade lavatories in April or May for quick toileting so experience in their use will be established for first grade.

Text and Library Books:

Leaf, Munro. *Health Can Be Fun.* New York: J.B. Lippincott Company, 1943, pp. 34-35.

Audio-Visual Materials:

Transparencies: "The Family."

4. *Concepts:* The wish for privacy in toilet procedures is a normal desire, not an expression of shame.

Learning Experiences: Capitalize on the informal, individual situation to explain this concept to the child.

5. *Concepts:* The child needs a wholesome attitude toward his body.

Learning Experiences: Through discussion with children, have these ideas brought out:

1. Healthy natural modesty is an outgrowth of one's control, dignity, and respect for self and others.
2. We show modesty by covering certain parts of the body because it shows respect for self and others.
3. The genitals are private, but not shameful.
4. If other persons ask to see or play with your private body parts, they are not very respectful of your body and permission should be denied.

6. *Concepts:* A child is brought into the world through love and affection, and his family loves him.

Learning Experiences: Children could cut pictures of family life from magazines and compile them in one big "family" book or on a bulletin board. Have children bring photos and snapshots of their own families to share and display in the room. You might read poetry expressing love and concern to the children.

"Little Brother".. Aileen Fisher
"Growing Up".. Author Unknown
"When a Fellow's Four".............................. Mary Jane Carr
"Five Years Old".................................... Marie Louise Allen

You might read selected poems of Marchette Chute and Dorothy Aldis as they pertain to childhood. Read stories of family life such as "The Little Family" and others. Use play corners to play family experiences.

Text and Library Books:

Teacher: Peterson, Eleanor. *Successful Living.* Chicago: Allyn and Bacon, 1959.

Aldis, Dorothy, *All Together.* New York: G.P. Putnam's Sons, 1952.

Brewton, Sara and John E. Brewton. *Birthday Candles Burning Bright.* New York: Macmillan Company, 1960.
Chute, Marchette. *Around and About.* New York: E.P. Dutton and Company, 1957.

7. *Concepts:* A child who feels secure in his role as a family member can adapt to changing situations.

Learning Experiences: Have children talk about ways they help at home. Pantomime scenes of family life where they are helping in some way.

Text and Library Books:

Burkhardt, Richard. *Our Family.* Chicago: Benefic Press, 1962.
Lenski, Lois. *Papa Small.* Garden City, New York: Doubleday, 1951.
Provus, Malcolm. *How Families Live Together.* Chicago: Benefic Press, 1963.

8. *Concepts:* The family helps shape personalities, develop values, habits, and attitudes toward life.

Learning Experiences: Have children use finger plays of family and home. Use songs that relate to family living.

Text and Library Books:

Carton, Lonnie. *Mommies.* New York: Random House, 1960.
Estes, Eleanor. *A Little Oven.* New York: Harcourt, Brace, 1955.
Lexau, Joanne M. *Every Day a Dragon.* New York: Harper, 1967.

Audio-Visual Materials:

Film: "We Play and Share Together," 11 minutes.
Sound Color Filmstrip: "Acceptance of Differences."

9. *Concepts:* The family provides love, companionship, security, and protection for all its members.

Learning Experiences: Show filmstrip "Keeping Busy." Talk with children about ways they may keep busy.

Text and Library Books:

Arbuthnot, May Hill. *Time for Poetry.* Chicago: Scott, Foresman Company, 1957. (selected poems, pp. 10-25)
Barber, Melvern. *The Different Twins.* New York: Lippincott, 1957.

Audio-Visual Materials:

Filmstrip: "Keeping Busy."

10. *Concepts:* The family guides individual members to understand, respect, and accept themselves.

Learning Experiences: Read stories of family life. Show and discuss the film, "Taking Care of Myself." Flannelgraph "families" may be used. The children can manipulate and dramatize with the figures. Show the filmstrip "Brothers and Sisters." Discuss with children the ideas presented. Have them tell the ways differences between brothers and sisters may be settled, as well as fun times they have together. Learn songs pertaining to families.

Text and Library Books:

Blomquist, David. *Daddy Is Home.* New York: Holt, Rinehart and Winston, Inc., 1963.
Eastman, Phillip D. *Are You My Mother?* New York: Random House, 1960.
Fehr, Howard F. *This Is My Family.* New York: Holt, Rinehart and Winston, Inc., 1963.
Guilfoile, Elizabeth. *Nobody Listens to Andrew.* Chicago: Follett Publishing Company, 1957.
Lenski, Lois. *Let's Play House.* New York: Walck, 1944.
Udry, Janice May. *Theodore's Parents.* New York: Lothrop Lee and Shepard Co., Inc., 1958.
Wittram, H.R. *My Little Brother.* New York: Holt, Rinehart and Winston, Inc., 1963.

Audio-Visual Materials:

Film: "Taking Care of Myself," 12 minutes.

Filmstrip: "Brothers and Sisters."

11. *Concepts:* The family provides necessary food, shelter, and material needs for all its members.

Learning Experiences: Make a mural of family life either with magazine pictures or ones that the children paint. In discussion bring out ideas of ways in which parents provide for us and ways in which we may help. Discuss the roles of grandmothers and grandfathers, especially if they live with the family.

Text and Library Books:

Teacher: Meilach, Dona Z. and Elias Mandel. *A Doctor Talks to Five to Eight Year Olds.* Chicago: Budlong Press Co., 5428 N. Virginia Avenue 60625, 1966.

12. *Concepts:* The family provides opportunities for the acceptance of responsibility and learning of respect for others.

Learning Experiences: Talk over with children what may happen if we don't accept responsibility. Have the children play scenes of caring for pets showing respect for others.

Text and Library Books:

Gruenberg, Sidonie Matsner. *The Wonderful Story of How You Were Born.* Garden City, New York: Doubleday and Company, Inc., 1959.

Audio-Visual Materials:

Filmstrip: "Growing Up."

13. *Concepts:* The family provides moral and spiritual values.

Learning Experiences: Show filmstrip "Our Family." Lead children to see that family living is a shared responsibility.

Text and Library Books:

Teacher: Anderson, Wayne J. *Design for Family Living.* Minneapolis: T.S. Denison and Company, Inc., 1965.

Lerrigo, Marion O. and Helen Southard. "Facts Aren't Enough." American Medical Association, 535 N. Dearborn St., Chicago, IL 60610.

_____. "Parent's Responsibility." American Medical Association, 535 N. Dearborn St., Chicago, IL 60610.

Rosenberg, Edward B. and Silas L. Warner. *The Pre-School Child's Learning Process.* Chicago: Budlong Press Co., 1967.

Buckley, Helen. *Grandfather and I.* New York: Lothrop, 1959.

_____. *Grandmother and I.* New York: Lothrop, 1961.

Audio-Visual Materials:

Filmstrip: "Our Family."

14. *Concepts:* Mother and father, as a result of love and affection, unite two cells to start the process of reproduction.

Learning Experiences: Children discuss the love of mother for father, father for mother, and their concern for the baby. In stories that children read together from readers, lead them to discover affection parents show for each other and for the baby. Read stories such as "Here Is the Ball" from the Junior Primer, Scott-Foresman and Company.

Text and Library Books:

Gruenberg, Sidonie. *The Wonderful Story of How You Were Born.*

Lerrigo, Marion O. and Helen Southard. "A Story About You." American Medical Association, 535 N. Dearborn St., Chicago, IL 60610, 1964.

15. *Concepts:* Prenatal growth and birth is a miraculous process.

Learning Experiences: Have children who have baby brothers and sisters share the experience of the way in which baby grows with care and love. Have children share experiences of ways in which the coming of the new baby has changed family life. Select slides that are suitable. Have children look at pictures in *Being Born* and *A Doctor Talks to Five to Eight Year Olds.* Write notes of welcome to send home at the birth of a baby brother or sister.

Draw pictures of the new baby. Read stories about new human babies. Read poetry of small babies:

"Little".. Dorothy Aldis
"The Twins" .... Elizabeth Madox Roberts
"Slippery".. Carl Sandburg

Text and Library Books:

Meilach and Mandel. *A Doctor Talks to Five to Eight Year Olds.*
Reed, Mary. *My First Book.* New York: Simon and Schuster, 1942.
Robinson, Helen M. *The New Guess Who.* Chicago: Scott, Foresman and Company, 1962, pp. 41-44.
Schlein, Miriam. *Laurie's New Brother.* Abelard, 1961.
Strain, Frances Bruce. *Being Born.* New York: Hawthorn, 1970.
Library: Arbuthnot. *Time for Poetry,* pp. 18, 22, 24.

Audio-Visual Materials:

Slides: "Family Life and Sex Education."

16. *Concepts:* The baby grows in a special place inside the mother's body called the uterus.

Learning Experiences: Use *Birth Atlas* to show the way in which the baby receives nourishment and protection.

Audio-Visual Materials:

Plates. Dickinson, Belskie. *Birth Atlas.* N.Y.: Maternity Center Association. (Library, 612.63 Dic).
"Life Before Birth" (*Life* Magazine Series).

17. *Concepts:* When the baby first starts to grow he doesn't look much like a baby, but very soon he has arms, legs, and is a miniature child.

Learning Experiences: When the question is asked regarding the appearance of the baby inside the uterus, the various pictures in the *Birth Atlas, A Doctor Talks to Five to Eight Year Olds, Being Born,* or the *Life Magazine* colored photographs may be viewed.

18. *Concepts:* The unborn baby moves and changes position while he is growing.

Learning Experiences: When the question or comment regarding movement arises, the above-listed references could be used to note the different positions.

19. *Concepts:* The baby is fed, breathes, and eliminates waste through the umbilical cord.

Learning Experiences: From the above-mentioned pictures (particularly the *Birth Atlas,* plates 6 and 7) the presence of the umbilical cord can be shown and discussed. Use *Birth Atlas* to show way in which baby is born. Read poetry about the baby.

"The Baby's Name" .... Tudor Jenks
"Six Weeks Old" .... Christopher Morley
"Hurry Tomorrow" .... Ivy O. Eastwick
"Little Phyllis" .... Kate Greenaway

Text and Library Books:

Ames, Gerald and Rose Wyler. *The Giant Golden Book of Biology.* New York: Golden Press, 1961.
Brewton and Brewton. *Birthday Candles Burning Bright.*
Ets, Marie Hall. *The Story of a Baby.* New York: Viking Press, 1939.

Audio-Visual Materials:

Dickinson, Belskie, *Birth Atlas.* N.Y.: Maternity Center Association.

20. *Concepts:* Human reproduction has a deep meaning.

Learning Experiences: Use animal study only as it relates to human beings and do not attempt to correlate this health material with animal units. Children and teacher collect pictures and develop a bulletin board on the ways in which human parents care for their children.

Text and Library Books:

Be aware of *My Weekly Reader* as a source of materials.

Arbuthnot. *Time for Poetry*, pp. 10-25.

Flack, Marjorie. *The New Pet.* Garden City, New York: Doubleday, 1943.

Audio-Visual Materials:

Note: Films related to animals and other science subjects such as
"Mother Hen's Family," "Happy Little Hamsters," "Kittens, Birth
and Growth," and "Vanishing Prairie" have not proven effective
in teaching first grade human sexuality concepts.

21. *Concepts:* Human babies are loved and cared for.

Learning Experiences: Draw pictures showing ways in which
human families love and care for babies. Bring pictures of selves as
babies; discuss change. Make scrapbooks or charts on ways human
families care for their young. Use stick or paper bag puppets to
create scenes of family living. Use play corner to play out family
care of baby.

Text and Library Books:

Teacher: Anderson. *Design for Family Living.*
Lerrigo and Southard. "Parent's Responsibility."
_____. "Facts Aren't Enough."
Peterson, Eleanor. *Successful Living.* Chicago: Allyn and Bacon,
1959.

Audio-Visual Materials:

Transparencies: "Living Things from Living Things."

22. *Concepts:* Humans are knit together in a family unit.

Learning Experiences: Have a mother bring baby to school. If
possible, have her bathe the baby. Make a book "All About Me"
stressing growth and change. Talk with children of the many kinds
of family groupings there are: mother, father and children; mother
and children; father and children; grandparents who care for
children; foster parents; adopted children; others.

Text and Library Books:

American Singer: "Rockaby Baby"—Book I.

Boardman, Eunice, *Exploring Music.* N.Y.: Holt, Rinehart and Winston, 1966. (Lullabies: "Go to Sleep," p. 127, "Mooki Mooki," p. 107, "Shoheen Sho," p. 144, "Sleep, Baby, Sleep," p. 133.

Audio-Visual Materials:

Transparencies: "Characteristics of Boys and Girls."

23. *Concepts:* Each sex identifies role with father or mother.

Learning Experiences: Discuss ways in which mother fulfills her role in the family. What is mother's role in the family? Child talks this over with mother. Discuss in class later, developing appreciation. Discuss ways in which father fulfills his role in the family. Discuss work role and familial responsibility of father, and ways children can help. Role play parts of mother and father in family situations. Create situations. Use props (apron, hat). Divide into groups of four or five. Read poetry of child identification with mother and father. Make bulletin board or mural showing ways in which mother and father are important to the family. Could be cut out of magazines, put in booklet form and saved. Read stories together about family living, both in library books and reading texts. Have child interpret the roles that mother and father play. How does father show his respect and love for mother? How does mother show her respect and love for father? Children relate experiences they have had in caring for younger sisters or brothers. This may be done in plays or in family picture drawings. Teacher may wish to relate to units on India and on Mexico. Read poetry: "Hiding"–Dorothy Aldis, "The Little Whistler"–Frances Frost, "Fun in a Garret"–Emma Dowd, "Picnic Day"–Rachel Field, "Away We Go"–Aileen Fisher.

Text and Library Books:

Teacher: Anderson. *Design for Family Living.*
Lerrigo and Southard. *Parent's Responsibility."*
_____. "Facts Aren't Enough."
Meilach and Mandel. *A Doctor Talks to Five to Eight Year Olds.*
Strain. *Being Born.*

Arbuthnot. *Time for Poetry.* "Neighborly," p. 10, "Andre," p. 13,
"Shop Windows," p. 14, "Smells," p. 14, "Walking," p. 15,
"Automobile Mechanics," p. 16, "Father," p. 17 (also pp. 229,
232-233, 236, 242, 243.)
Bulla, Clyde Robert. *Ghost Town Treasure.* New York: Crowell,
1957.
Haywood, Carolyn. *B Is for Betsy.* New York: Harcourt, Brace,
Jovanovich, 1968.
_____. *Betsy's Little Star.* New York: Morrow, 1950.
_____. *Little Eddie.* New York: Morrow, 1947.
_____. *Mixed-Up Twins.* New York: Morrow, 1952.
Reyher, Becky. *My Mother Is the Most Beautiful Woman in the
World.* New York: Lothrop, 1945.

Audio-Visual Materials:

Films: "Appreciating Our Parents," 10 minutes, b/w.
"The Family."
"A Family of India," 16 minutes.
"Health and Happiness of the Family."
"The Story of Pablo, Mexican Boy," 22 minutes.
"Taking Care of Myself," 12 minutes.

24. *Concepts:* Society often imposes different roles for girls and
boys.

Learning Experiences: Help children to see that there is some
degree of maleness and femaleness in each of us. "For example,
when a situation arises that causes a boy or man to cry from pain
or frustration or in sympathy, he is not acting like a girl, but is
only exhibiting a sensitivity common to all persons" *(Journal of
School Health).* Roles of mother and father may overlap. Father
may care for children while mother goes out to work.

Text and Library Books:

Teacher: The Journal of School Health, May, 1967. American
School Health Association, pp. 47, 48.
Beim, Jerrold. *The Smallest Boy in the Class.* New York: William
Morrow and Company, 1949.

de Angeli, Marguerite. *The Empty Barn.* Philadelphia: Westminster Press, 1966.

Yashima, Mitsu and Taro Yashima. *Crow Boy.* New York: Viking Press, 1955.

25. *Concepts:* Choice and interest should determine our work.

Learning Experiences: Discuss with children types of workers they like: astronauts, baseball players, etc. The world of work is wide with opportunity for girls and boys. Discuss "Why can both men and women be fire fighters, nurses, etc.?"

Text and Library Books:

Pamphlets: Ten pamphlets on self-concept can be obtained from Child Study Association of America, Crowell Publishers, 9 East 8th St., New York, N.Y. 10023.

26. *Concepts:* The child is developing a concept of his role in society.

Learning Experiences: Have child do various classroom chores in which he finds satisfaction. Teacher should arrange for each child to be a leader at some time. Find ways in which individuals may relate to the larger unit of the school: student council activities, special projects. Discuss leadership role in out-of-school activities. Use songs from music books that relate to child activities.

Text and Library Books:

Suggested Music: Boardman, *Exploring Music,* Book 2. "After School," p. 13, "Poor Lolotte," p. 15, "The Animal Fair," pp. 16-17, "Morning Song," p. 97.

Audio-Visual Materials:

Film: "Getting Along with Others," 11 minutes.

27. *Concepts:* Each person must discover and develop his own self-concept.

Learning Experiences: Determine, through discussion, the interests and activities of each child. Provide opportunities for children to bring hobbies for display and, when possible, take part in favorite activities. Provide for a positive evaluation period of what each achieved that day. Ask: "What did you like best about school?" Put on a hobby show. Sharing: Tell about selves—what you like, what you do. Seek out library and reading text stories that may interpret child's role in society. Have a "Barrel of Happy Thoughts" (glass jar) where teacher records children's positive statements of the strengths and capabilities of their classmates as they observe them in work and play (Ex.: "Janice shared her jump rope with the first graders."). Help child make a booklet containing thoughts on:

What I Like About myself
What I Don't Like About Myself
How I Can Improve Myself

Put books out to start this section. Correlate with language arts. Let each child keep a personal, secret notebook and set aside a few minutes each day to record something in this notebook. Items such as: What made me happy today? sad? angry? Did I do something nice for someone? Did someone do something nice for me? Have children make a book "Happy Thoughts." Discuss feelings and experiences that are pleasant and unpleasant. Encourage children to use puppets as an outlet for their feelings of anger and frustration. Use puppets also in situations of positive self worth. Discuss storybook characters with which the children are familiar in terms of the following: (may be used in reading discussion)

Why do I like this character?
Is there anything I do not like about him?
Why would he be fun to play with?
Can I see any characteristics of mine in this character?

Text and Library Books:

Authors who help develop good self-concept through their writings:

Jerrold Beim, Emma Brock, Pearl S. Buck, Clyde Robert Bulla,
Marie Hall Ets, Eleanor F. Lattimore, Miriam Mason.

Ayars, James S. *Happy Birthday, Mom.* New York: Abelard-
Schuman, 1963.

Beim, Jerrold. *Jay's Big Job.* New York: Morrow, 1957.

_____. *Swimming Hole.* New York: Morrow, 1951.

_____. *Taming of Toby.* New York: Morrow, 1953.

Brown, Myra Berry. *Birthday Boy.* New York: Watts, Inc., 1963.

Ets, Marie Hall. *Bad Boy, Good Boy.* New York: Crowell, 1967.

Zolotov, Charlotte. *Big Brother.* New York: Harper, 1960.

Audio-Visual Materials:

Film: "What to Do About Upset Feelings," 11 minutes.
Sound Color Filmstrip: "Learning to Be Unselfish."
Transparencies: "Characteristics of Boys and Girls."

28. *Concepts:* Our body has many complex parts.

Learning Experiences: Use oral review to list parts of the body
children already know, bringing out child's knowledge of genital
areas. This may be done on a one-to-one basis.

29. *Concepts:* We keep our bodies clean.

Learning Experiences: Discuss cleanliness as a necessary daily
activity.

30. *Concepts:* One of the reasons to keep vulva and penis clean is
that each of these is a part of the urinary system.

Learning Experiences: Review parts of the body that we keep
clean, being certain to include penis, scrotum, and vulva.

Audio-Visual Materials:

Transparencies: "Characteristics of Boys and Girls."
"The Family."

31. *Concepts:* The external genitalia are a part of the reproductive
system.

Learning Experiences: Show pictures of statue by Verrocchio, and *David* by Michelangelo.

Text and Library Books:

Meilach and Mandel. *A Doctor Talks to Five to Eight Year Olds,* pp. 21-27; pictures— *David* by Michelangelo, p. 25, and statue by Verrocchio, p. 47.

Audio-Visual Materials:

Slides: David by Michelangelo from *A Doctor Talks to Five to Eight Year Olds* (p. 25). Statue by Verrocchio from *A Doctor Talks to Five to Eight Year Olds* (p. 47).

32. *Concepts:* Purpose in reproduction: The penis deposits sperm into the vagina. The scrotum holds the testicles. Testicles produce sperm. Vulva is the opening to let sperm in and serves to let the baby out.

Learning Experiences: Teacher gives statements that tell function of each body part. Develop and maintain a learning climate where children will feel free to ask questions.[3]

---

[3]*Guide for Teaching Health in the Area of Human Relations and Sexuality,* K-6, *8 and 11.*

CHAPTER 6 *The Curriculum for the Middle Grades*

Levels of Psychosexual Development

The Nine- to Ten-Year-Old

Boys and girls of this age are fairly well-rooted in reality. They have more or less come to terms with themselves, their parents, their groups, and their school. Their knowledge grows daily, and their interests increase rapidly. Extremely curious about everything, they want and are ready for facts. Not yet mature sexually themselves, they are nevertheless interested in the facts of life. Because they are preadolescent and not yet emotionally involved on a personal basis, they accept aspects of sex education as they do the facts about all body functions and other matters.

Generally, each sex is indifferent to or even hostile to the other one. It is an age for teasing and bickering, name-calling, "bad" language, and "gang secrets" like signs, passwords, and codes. In striving for individual identity and the beginning of independence, boys and girls may regard the opinions of their friends as more important than those of their parents.

Girls may move ahead toward maturity more quickly at this stage and become extremely interested in menstruation, conception, and childbirth. Boys are especially curious and eager for sexual knowledge and usually obtain it in magazines, medical books, or from older adolescents. There are sometimes secret discussions and speculations about sexual activities.

Although still favoring their own sex and still somewhat awkward and uneasy with girls, boys are beginning to show an interest in the other sex, but teasing and more aggressive behavior mask any overt sexual interest. As both boys and girls grow toward puberty, they begin to shift back and forth between wanting to be grown up and wishing for childhood attentions. This conflict gives rise to some reactions of unruliness, disorderliness, and stubbornness, if not downright disobedience. There are mood changes as both boys and girls look forward, some with fear and apprehension and some with welcome anticipation, to their on-coming puberty. Knowledge related to family living and sex education is important so that these young people may develop positive attitudes toward their own sexuality.

It is necessary for youngsters at this age to gain deeper understanding of their physical and psychosocial growth. They are deeply concerned with what will happen to them as individuals and require knowledge of these specifics prior to their own sexual maturation. In today's society they are constantly exposed to a variety of information and misinformation about sexual matters; hence they are in great need of factual data.[1]

OUTLINE

"Understanding of and Respect for Reproductive Organs"

A. Each person needs to be able to locate and identify his reproductive organs.

    1. The male reproductive organs are generally outside the body.
       a. One must use correct terminology.
       b. One must understand the general functions of the reproductive system.
       c. One must appreciate the wonder of the reproductive functions.

    2. The female reproductive organs are generally inside the body.
       a. One must use correct terminology.

---

[1]"Family Living Including Sex Education Guide," N.Y.C. Bureau of Curriculum Development, Board of Education, New York City, series 1969-1970.

b. One must understand the general function of the reproductive system.

c. One must appreciate the wonder of the reproductive functions.

B. Each person must understand the danger of injury to his reproductive organs.

   1. Kicking others in the groin and pelvic area may injure the reproductive organs.

      a. In the male there may be permanent injury to the testicles.

      b. In the female there may be damage to the vulva.

   2. Hitting or kicking in the abdomen of a female can cause permanent damage to the developing uterus and ovaries.

   3. Hitting the breast of a female can cause permanent damage to the developing mammary glands.

C. Each person must recognize and take precautionary measures against invasions of his personal privacy by persons other than his parents or medical personnel.

   1. Molesters may be stranger, friend, or relative.

   2. There are many advantages in being with companions in public.

   3. A lack of modesty invites problems. This is especially true in public facilities.

"The Need for Families as a Basic Unit of Human Life"

D. The family is a basic unit of human living.

E. The family brings children into the world and prepares them for adulthood.

   1. It helps them in problem solving.

   2. It helps them make adjustments to life.

F. The family provides love, security, care, and protection.

G. The family provides moral and spiritual guidance.

H. The family furnishes values and ideals.

I. The family develops a self-concept within each member.

J. The family preserves its heritage (the values, culture, and religious beliefs).

K. The family fosters consideration and sensitivity to feelings of others.

L. The family helps the child relate to society and to the world community.

M. The family provides sex education.
1. It answers questions regarding maturational changes.
   a. There are changes in height due to the pituitary gland.
      (1) Classmates are no longer the same size.
      (2) The girls are getting taller than the boys.
      (3) The change in boys will come later.
   b. There is a difference in size and build from child to child.
      (1) Some of this change is due to heredity.
      (2) Some of this change may be due to nutrition.
   c. These changes follow a pattern.
      (1) The pattern depends upon heredity.
      (2) The pattern develops individuality.
2. It provides opportunity for the child to consult with his parents.
3. It helps develop within each child the responsibility to master his own body machinery.[2]

---

[2]*Guide for Teaching Health in the Area of Human Relations and Sexuality K-6, 8 and 11.* Independent School District No. 77, Mankato, Minnesota 56001, 1968. Used by permission.

The Curriculum

Grades 3 and 4

1. *Concepts:* The location and correct terminology for our reproductive organs is necessary for better understanding and respect.

Learning Experiences: Review the location and proper identification of all the organs of reproduction listed in the vocabulary. This would be followed by a review of the function of each of these.

Text and Library Books:

Gruenberg, Sidonie. *The Wonderful Story of How You Were Born.* Garden City, N.Y.: Doubleday, 1959.
Lerrigo, Marion O. and Helen Southard. "A Story About You." Chicago: American Medical Association, 1964, pp. 40-41.

Audio-Visual Materials:

Slide: David by Michelangelo from *A Doctor Talks to Five to Eight Year Olds,* p. 25.
(Films related to animals and other subject matter areas have not proved effective in teaching these third-grade human sexuality concepts.)

2. *Concepts:* All discussions and learning should lead to a more wholesome attitude on the part of the child toward his reproductive organs.

Learning Experiences: Emphasize the future role of children as good fathers and mothers, showing that the intention is to help them grow into well-adjusted adults. Emphasis should be maintained on the positive aspects of these issues.

3. *Concepts:* Our reproductive organs are vulnerable to damage during accident or fighting. Therefore, we should be aware of these dangers and learn how to protect ourselves from them.

Learning Experiences: Before the unit or during the introduction of the unit a question box may be placed on the teacher's desk where pupils may drop their questions. Perhaps a lead question could be placed in the box such as, "What do you feel are some dangers to your reproductive organs?" These questions would then be answered in the class discussion, possibly helping to lead into more questions. This concept may be discussed when the boys begin to grab each other in the groin area. List possible sources of danger to the reproductive organs such as a kick or blow to the testicles or breasts and have the children discuss the possible damage that might come of this. Discuss bars, hurdles, bicycles, as possible other dangerous agents in injuring testicles. Have a discussion covering the dangers of playing tackle football without proper protective equipment. After it has been made clear where the danger exists, the teacher should point out the proper way to play, making the emphasis that good safety habits may make a healthier adulthood possible. Using a diagram of the reproductive organs, show how a kick might affect them, projecting some problems that may arise, cautioning them to avoid this situation by safe play.

4. *Concepts:* We should take care not to damage the reproductive organs of others, either in jest or in anger.

Learning Experiences: Set up role-playing activities where safe and acceptable ways of venting one's anger are portrayed. Project an unfinished situational story and have each child give or write his own ending. Use demonstrations showing how to protect oneself from a groin kick. Discuss how groin kicks are used in the movies and T.V., covering how the stunt men practice not really kicking in the groin, but making it appear that way; and how they wear a protective guard to prevent accidents. Have children interested in sports report on protective gear worn by professional athletes.

Text and Library Books:

Teacher: Anderson, Wayne. *Design for Family Living.* Minneapolis: T.S. Denison and Company, 1964, pp. 215-216.

Starr, Helen and James Fox. *The Teaching Resource Manual in Human Sexuality Education for Preschool, Kindergarten, and Primary Grades.* Minneapolis: T.A.M.A., 1967, pp. 17 and 31.

5. *Concepts:* We should not allow or encourage others to touch our reproductive organs.

Learning Experiences: Hold a class discussion pointing out how immodest dress, dressing habits, or improper sitting posture would invite problems with a person who does not understand his or her sex role (sexual deviates). Discuss appropriate dress. Use role playing to show the different aspects of not accepting rides, candy, money, and other forms of bribery from a stranger or acquaintance. The child may jot the license plate number on the ground. Puppets may also be used to show different ways in which strangers may entice a child close to or into his car or house (such as asking directions, telling the child to take him to a destination, offering candy, rides, or money). A policeman may talk to the children. Class discussion could lead to the construction of a chart of guidelines or set of safety rules on the subject of dealing with strangers, noting that children should not play in empty buildings, alleys, or lonely places. Point out that most people are friendly and that children should be guided by parental permission before accepting gifts from people, or going with friends of the family or friendly strangers. (Please do not tell of or describe acts of sex perversion, or use a warning approach in teaching this concept.) When the time of year for door-to-door solicitations comes around, suggest to children that it would be better for their safety if they went in pairs. Advise that in attending movies, they go with others. Suggest that if somebody tries to touch them, to leave their seat. Tell the usher or person in charge. Never go with a stranger to the washroom or for a ride.

Text and Library Books:

Teacher: David, Lester. "How Parents Fight Sex Crimes Against Children," *Good Housekeeping,* July, 1966.

6. *Concepts:* The family brings the child into the world and prepares him for adulthood by helping him meet problems and make adjustments to life.

Learning Experiences: Establish recognition and meaning for the vocabulary contained in the outline.

Have the children discuss the ongoing love of family for each other from generation to generation. Write an expression of family love and feeling.

Read aloud to the children *The Beech Tree* by Pearl Buck and have the class discuss its implications.

Conduct role playing situations growing out of "Happy Feelings Are Important" from *Going on Ten.*

Text and Library Books:

Bauer, W.W., et al. *Going on Ten.* Chicago: Scott-Foresman and Co., 1962, pp. 39-41, 121-130.
Buck, Pearl. *The Beech Tree.* New York: John Day Co., 1955.
Mead, Margaret. *People and Places.* New York: World, 1959.
Mead, Margaret, and Ken Keyman. *The Family.* New York: Macmillan, 1965.
Seymour, Alta. *The Christmas Stove.* New York: Wilcox, 1951.
Underhill, Ruth M. *First Came the Family.* New York: Morrow, 1958.

Audio-Visual Materials:

Sound Color Filmstrips: "Getting Along with Our Family."
"Learning How to Be Liked."
"Learning to Be Forgiving."
"Learning to Make Friends."
"Learning to Use Money Wisely."

7. *Concepts:* The family provides love, security, care and protection.

Learning Experiences: Have children discuss their favorite book family such as the family in the books by Laura Ingalls Wilder, showing how this family interacts.

Discuss these questions: (this could be done in small groups)
How can parents show love for children?
How can children show love for parents?
How can brothers and sisters show love for one another?

Text and Library Books:

Favorite Families: Caudill, Rebecca. *Happy Little Family.* Holt, Rinehart and Winston, 1963.

Wilder, Laura Ingalls. *Little House in the Big Woods.* Harper and
Row, 1953.
‗‗‗‗‗‗ *Little House on the Prairie.* Harper and Row, 1953.
‗‗‗‗‗‗ *On the Banks of Plum Creek.* Harper and Row, 1953.

8. *Concepts:* One of many different combinations may form a
family grouping.

Learning Experiences: Dramatize scenes where families provide
love, security, care and protection.
Arrange a bulletin board on the different ages possible in a
family—"A Family Affair." Example: mother-child, father-child,
family-new baby, young family, middle-aged family, grandparents,
foster, adopted, others. Discuss how to reconcile differences with
each other and with families.
Read poetry together such as "Beach Fire" by Frances Frost.
Have children tell of similar experiences.

Text and Library Books:

Arbuthnot, May Hill. *Time for Poetry.* Chicago: Scott-Foresman
and Co., 1959, p. 231, selected poems, pp. 10-25.
Armer, Laura. *Waterless Mountain.* New York: McKay, 1931.
Brink, Carol Ryrie. *Caddie Woodlawn.* New York: Macmillan Co.,
1959.
Chastain, Madys Lee. *Fripsey Summer.* New York: Harcourt Brace
and Co., 1953.
Estes, Eleanor. *The Hundred Dresses.* New York: Harcourt Brace
Jovanovich, 1974.
‗‗‗‗‗‗ *The Moffats.* New York: Harcourt Brace Jovanovich,
1968.

Audio-Visual Materials:
Sound Color Filmstrip: "Working Together in the Family."

9. *Concepts:* The family provides moral and spiritual guidance.
The family furnishes values and ideals.

Learning Experiences: Role play family situations in which
moral and spiritual values are upheld. Use books such as *A Penny's*

Worth of Character by Jesse Stuart, and short stories in reading series where values are recognized as in the Benjamin West stories by Marguerite Henry.

Text and Library Books:

Robinson, Helen M. *Ventures.* Chicago: Scott-Foresman and Company, 1965, pp. 248-256.
Stuart, Jesse. *A Penny's Worth of Character.* N.Y.: McGraw-Hill Book Company, 1961.

10. *Concepts:* Dress appropriately for the occasion.

Learning Experiences: Discuss proper dress for answering the door at home or for entertaining friends. Why is it more acceptable for a young child than for an adult to appear in pajamas? What is appropriate dress for the place and occasion?

Text and Library Books:

Gates, Doris. *Blue Willow.* N.Y.: The Viking Press, 1969.

11. *Concepts:* The family helps develop the self-concept of each member.

Learning Experiences: Discuss with children the changing roles of parents in our culture. The following are examples:

More mothers are outside the home adding to family income and taking part in church and civic affairs.
The father may be geographically separated from the family—on the road, in service, etc. His work may be in a computerized world and of a nature not easily understood by the family.

Have the child explain his role as a family member.
Read the poem "Me" by Walter de la Mare. Have the children create personal expressions of "me" either in poetry or prose.

Text and Library Books:

Byrd, Neilson, Moore. *Health,* Second edition. River Forest, Ill.: Laidlaw Bros., 1966, pp. 94-97.
Teacher: Peterson, Eleanor, *Successful Living.* Chicago: Allyn and Bacon, 1959.

Audio-Visual Materials:

Transparencies: "The Health and Happiness of the Family."

12. *Concepts:* The family preserves the heritage of values, culture, and religious beliefs.

Learning Experiences: Correlate with social studies using background of knowledge of Israel and other family patterns and cultures. Emphasize traditions and mores.

Have children seek out background of their own inheritance.

Have children write of some special observance or custom in their own families—birthday, Christmas, or others.

Show filmstrip "Family Fun." Have children discuss the types of values this family holds. Have children illustrate a surprise planned for their own family members.

Text and Library Books:

Buck, Pearl S. *The Chinese Children Next Door.* N.Y.; John Day Co., 1952.

Bulla, Clyde R. *Indian Hill.* N.Y.: Crowell, 1963.

Clark, Ann Nolan. *Little Navajo Bluebird.* N.Y.: Viking, 1943.

de Angeli, Marguerite. *Bright April.* N.Y.: Doubleday, 1946.

Lawson, Robert. *They Were Strong and Good.* N.Y.: Viking, 1940.

Lenski, Lois. *Cotton in My Sack.* Philadelphia: Lippincott, 1949.

Taylor, Sydney. *All-Of-A-Kind Family* (series). Chicago: Follett Publishing Co., 1951.

Audio-Visual Materials:

Filmstrip: "Family Fun."

13. *Concepts:* The family fosters consideration and sensitivity to others such as understanding feelings of jealousy regarding a new baby.

Learning Experiences: Show film "Family Team Work." Analyze ways in which the family fosters consideration and sensitivity to others. Here are some of the ideas from the film for discussion:

Older sister is kind to younger brothers and sisters.

Each child contributes to the welfare of the family. List ways. Family is involved in a common interest.

Their day includes work and play. Evening is experienced as a family group.

Have children find out some of the things they did before they were old enough to remember. How is the new baby like they were?

Use transparencies such as "Individual Health and Family Life" for discussing how each situation affects the family.

Text and Library Books:

Buck, Pearl S. *Welcome Child.* N.Y.: John Day Co., 1963.
Duncan, Lois. *Giving Away Suzanne.* N.Y.: Dodd, Mead, 1963.
Scott, Sally. *Judy's Baby.* N.Y.: Harcourt, Brace and Co., 1949.

Send for: Books for Friendship, Anti-Defamation League, American Friends, 160 N. 15 St., Philadelphia, PA.

Audio-Visual Materials:

Transparencies: "Individual Health and Family Life."

14. *Concepts:* The family helps the child relate to society and the world community.

Learning Experiences: Lead children to discover that basic needs are the same no matter what the cultural setting.

Establish pen pal correspondence, especially with children of other lands.

Use United Nations material, World Health Organization, and UNICEF as learning and participation experiences.

Bring in college or high school students or community people of different ethnic backgrounds to speak on home and family. Have them stay for lunch with the children.

Learn folk songs and folk dances of other lands. This may be part of music and physical education.

Text and Library Books:

Check with Junior Red Cross for establishing pen pals. You may also contact:

UNA USA, 345 E. 46th St., N.Y., N.Y. 10017.

UNA of Minnesota, 208 Times Annex, Minneapolis, Minn. 55401.

U.S. Committee for UNICEF, UNA, 345 E. 46th St., N.Y., N.Y. 10017.

Music Texts: Boardman, Eunice. *Exploring Music.* N.Y.: Holt, Rinehart and Winston, 1966.

Thomas, Edith L. *The Whole World Singing.* N.Y.: Friendship Press (475 Riverside Drive, 10027).

Folk Songs of Other Countries: Lewiston, Mina. *Faces Looking Up.* N.Y.: Harper and Bros., 1960.

Teacher: Anderson. *Design for Family Living.*

15. *Concepts:* The function of the family is to answer questions on sex education. Parents want to help.

Learning Experiences: Discuss with children ways in which they could recognize when their parents want to help them.

Text and Library Books:

Teacher Source Material: Lerrigo, Marion O. and Michael Cassidy. *A Doctor Talks to Nine to Twelve Year Olds.* Chicago: Budlong Press Co., 1969.

Strain, Frances. *Being Born.* N.Y.: Hawthorn, 1970.

Series of publications by Marion Lerrigo and Helen Southard: "A Story About You," "Parent's Responsibility," "Facts Aren't Enough," "Finding Yourself." All published by the American Medical Association, 535 N. Dearborn St., Chicago, IL 60610.[3]

---

[3] *Guide for Teaching Health in the Area of Human Relations and Sexuality, K-6, 8 and 11.*

CHAPTER 7   *The Curriculum for the Intermediate Grades*

Levels of Psychosexual Development

The Eleven- to Thirteen-Year-Old

The eleven- to thirteen-year-old is embarking upon the struggle to develop a relatively autonomous self in preparation for independent adulthood. In so doing he seeks to control his dependence on his parents by transferring some of the emotional attachments he has to them and to others outside of his immediate family. His pal relationships with peers of his own sex acquire greater significance as they meet his needs for new attachments. As he realizes his continuing and inevitable dependence on parents and teachers, he often experiences conflict and anxiety. Consequently, he may tend to withdraw from the adults with whom he had previously enjoyed close attachments. Irritable, defiant behavior may support this withdrawal. On the other hand, crushes on adults and admiration of popular figures are likely to emerge as less threatening forms of attachment to adults.

During this period, the youngster tries to establish his identity further by working toward his own code of moral and ethical values. In order to do so, he wrestles with absolutes of right and wrong and is acutely aware of inconsistencies in the behavior of others, especially in the behavior of the significant adults in his life.

At this age the youngster begins to examine role definitions. In this way he gathers data upon which to base his emerging

137

self-identity. He is concerned with many questions: How should a husband and wife relate to each other? How should siblings deal with each other? How should a mother or father act toward a boy or girl? The "shoulds" and ideal models that result often give rise to anxious doubting and criticism of self and others. Youngsters at this age are often reassured by being helped to understand the varieties of human encounter.

While sexual and aggressive drives are just beginning to emerge, they may be frightening to the early adolescent. Since bodies are changing, anxious self-scrutiny focuses on fear of abnormality. Girls are self-conscious about breast development or lack of it. They worry about menstruation. Boys are concerned about their strength and height. Very often size and physical development determine choices of companions and become a basis for self-esteem.

Some young people are very much concerned about masturbation and the feelings of guilt that frequently accompany this behavior. Opportunities to discuss the changes that may be taking place within themselves with informed, understanding adults are most important.

The early adolescent often relates inconsistently to adult authority. He questions, challenges, idolizes, is hypercritical and dependent, often all at the same time. He is very interested in aspects of human behavior such as manliness, womanliness, motherhood, etc., and seeks to apply these conceptualizations to himself and to others close to him. As the teacher helps him to find a realistic view of behavior, his own and others, he is less moved to prove himself in extreme ways. It is important to help him think issues through for himself, especially since he is intolerant of directive absolutes, and is ready to establish an independently integrated value system. While he is still strongly influenced by adult opinion, he is even more interested in the opinions of his peers, so that classroom discussions are especially relevant at this time. Frank discussion of sexual matters produces considerable anxiety and embarrassment as well as curiosity, hence the jokes and snickering. However, facts about bodily changes and role behavior hold the attention of the early adolescent and are important at this time. Youngsters of this age need to be reassured about the normality of sexual feelings and helped to establish controls. The most important challenge to the teacher is to reinforce the eleven- to thirteen-year-old's self-esteem in his search for competence in preparing himself to deal with the issue of adulthood.[1]

OUTLINE—Intermediate Grades

"The Anatomy and Physiology of the Human Reproductive System"

A. There are glands that affect your growth.

    1. The pituitary is an endocrine gland.
        a. It is located at the base of the brain.
        b. It is about the size of a small cherry.
        c. It controls the growth patterns of the body.
    2. The testicles secrete a hormone.
    3. The ovaries secrete a hormone.

B. All parts of the reproductive system have a definite function.

    1. There are many female organs.
        a. The vulva is the region around the external opening of the reproductive system.
        b. The vagina is the birth canal.
        c. The uterus provides protection and nourishment for the embryo and fetus.
        d. The Fallopian tubes carry the ovum to the uterus.
        e. The ovaries produce ova.
    2. There are many male organs.
        a. The penis discharges semen and urine.
        b. The urethra is the tube that carries semen and urine.
        c. The prostate gland secretes a fluid discharged with the semen.
        d. The seminal vesicles store semen.
        e. The vas deferens carries sperm.
        f. The testicles produce sperm.

---

[1] "Family Living Including Sex Education Guide," N.Y.C. Bureau of Curriculum Development, Board of Education, New York City, series 1969-1970.

(1) Sperm are expelled during a nocturnal emission.

(2) Sperm may be expelled during masturbation.

C. There are normal processes of the reproductive system.

    1. Menstruation is a normal process wherein blood and tissue are passed from the body.

    2. Nocturnal emissions (wet dreams) are a normal process wherein semen is passed from the body.

Correct terminology for teachers to use in discussing these concepts:

glands, pituitary, testicles, ovaries, gonads, hormones, vulva, vagina, uterus, menstruation, Fallopian tube, penis, urethra, prostate, seminal vesicles, vas deferens, nocturnal emissions, masturbation, ejaculation, womb, anatomy, endocrine glands physiology, puberty, spermatozoa, semen, urinate, urine, void.

"Human Reproduction"

D. Male sex cells are produced.

    1. Sperm are minute cells with heads and active tails.

    2. The sperm follow a pathway out of the body.

       a. They start in the testes.

       b. The vas deferens is a tube through which they travel.

       c. The seminal vesicles store the sperm.

       d. The urethra is a passageway to the outside of the body.

       e. The penis is erect during ejaculation.

E. The sperm journeys to meet the ovum during mating.

    1. The sperm travel through the vagina.

    2. The sperm travel through the uterus.

    3. The sperm enter the Fallopian tubes.

F. Female sex cells are produced.

    1. The ova are round-shaped cells.

    2. The ovum follows a pathway after ovulation.

       a. The ovum leaves the ovary.

       b. The ovum travels through the Fallopian tube.

G. The miracle of life begins when the sperm and ovum meet.

1. Fertilization is the union of a sperm and an ovum.
   a. These two cells form a new life.
   b. The completed cell is called a fertilized cell.
2. The many factors of heredity begin their effect immediately.
   a. The two parent cells contain all the substances that make a child look like his ancestors.
   b. The substances that control heredity are called chromosomes.
      (1) There are 23 chromosome chains with parental characteristics in each parent cell.
      (2) There is also one chromosome to determine sex.
   c. There are many genes to each chromosome.
3. Promiscuity may lead to unwanted children.

H. Prenatal growth occurs in the uterus.

1. The embryo attaches itself to the lining of the uterus.
2. The placenta and umbilical cord system develop.
   a. Nourishment and oxygen come from the mother.
   b. Waste materials are carried off.
   c. The blood systems of the child and the mother never mingle.
3. The internal parts of the body grow.
   a. The heart develops.
   b. The brain develops.
   c. The stomach develops.
   d. The lungs develop.
4. The external parts of the body grow.
   a. The head with eyes grows.
   b. The body with arms and legs grows.
5. The fetus grows for about nine months (gestation period).
   a. It becomes about 7 pounds in weight.
   b. It becomes about 20 inches in length.
   c. It is suspended in a fluid, inside a sac.
      (1) This protects it from bumps.
      (2) This keeps the temperature even.

I. Birth occurs.

1. The muscles of the uterus begin to gently contract.
2. The cervix opens.
3. The baby comes down through the vagina.
4. The doctor may assist.
    a. He may help the baby out.
    b. He cuts the umbilical cord.

Correct terminology to be used by teacher in discussing concepts:

sperm cell, testes, vas deferens, seminal vesicles, urethra, penis, vagina, uterus, ovum, ovary, Fallopian tube, fertilization, heredity, chromosomes, genes, culture, egg cell, nucleus, dominant trait, recessive trait, placenta, umbilical, navel, nourishment, embryo, oxygen, internal, external, fetus, womb, birth canal, cervix, gestation, mating, ovulation, sexual promiscuity, protoplasm, obstetrician, semen[2]

[2]*Guide for Teaching Health in the Area of Human Relations and Sexuality K-6, 8 and 11.* Independent School District No. 77, Mankato, Minnesota 56001, 1968. Used by permission.

The Curriculum
Grades 5 and 6

1. *Concepts:* The pituitary gland affects your growth.

Learning Experiences: Bring a large pea or small cherry to class to illustrate the the size of the pituitary gland. Compare the effects of the pituitary gland on boys and girls. Boys could study and report the effect on boys; girls study and report the effect on girls. Have the class as a whole discuss the role of the pituitary gland on the range of height among their age group. (Chart on p. 251 of *About Yourself.*) Hold a discussion regarding growth spurts and plateaus and how the youngster fits into the pattern. Have children select a panel to discuss the pros and cons of why the pituitary might be called the master gland. Construct an outline of the skull on the bulletin board with a small circle in the relative position of the pituitary gland. Radiating lines from the position of the pituitary would list the effects of the pituitary gland on boys (lines on one side of the skull) and girls (lines on the other side). Discuss the role of the pituitary gland in the growth of dwarfs and giants. Collect magazine pictures for bulletin board display, illustrating differences in size and physique among adults. Hold a discussion, comparing individuals within the class regarding size and physique among its members. If this is done, care should be taken to assure a good attitude on the part of the persons being selected for comparison.

Text and Library Books:

Teacher: Lerrigo, Marion and Helen Southard. "Facts Aren't Enough." Chicago: American Medical Association, 1962, p. 38.
Student: Bauer, W.W. *et al. About Yourself.* Glenview, Ill.: Scott, Foresman and Co., 1962, pp. 246-252.
Byrd, Oliver E. *et al. Health Five.* River Forest, Ill.: Laidlaw Brothers, 1966, pp. 173-174.
———— *Your Health.* River Forest, Ill.: Laidlaw Brothers, 1960, pp. 174-175.
Cooley, Donald G. "Hormones: Your Body's Chemical Rousers," Part I, *Today's Health,* Vol. XL, No. 11, November 1962, pp. 28-33, 72-74.

_____ "Hormones: Your Body's Chemical Rousers," Part II, *Today's Health,* Vol. XL, No. 12, December 1962, pp. 28-31, 86-87.

Hofstein, Sadie and W. W. Bauer. *The Human Story—Facts on Birth, Growth, Reproduction.* Glenview, Ill.: Scott-Foresman and Co., 1967, pp. 10-11.

Lerrigo, Marion and Helen Southard. "Facts Aren't Enough," p. 38.

Audio-Visual Materials:

Transparencies: "Endocrine System" from T.A.M.A. Kit No. II *(Human Sexuality Education, Upper Elementary Grades),* Teaching Aids Medically Authenticated, 608 Second Avenue S., Minneapolis, Minn. 55402, 1968.

"Human Growth and Development" (male and female divisions) from T.A.M.A. Kit No. II (A-V media kit).

Sound Color Filmstrip: "Life Begins: Human Reproduction."

Bulletin Board: Construct a bulletin board similar to the one listed in the Learning Experiences section to give students a chance to study these concepts at their leisure.

2. *Concepts:* Knowing the size and location of each organ in the reproductive system helps us understand more about it.

Learning Experiences: Using a diagram of the human body, a location should be made, by the student or the teacher, for each of the parts of the reproductive system. In order to assure correct individual concepts, have each student make his own individual drawings or diagrams of the reproductive systems for his own notebook. Labeling parts of duplicate diagrams has not proven an effective teaching device. (When children draw their own diagrams, it is best to send them home as part of a unit booklet rather than as individual papers.) A mature group could make large butcher paper outlines of the human body (a male on one end of the bulletin board, and a female on the other), making construction paper outlines of various organs, identifying them and putting them in the proper place. The showing of the film "Girl to Woman" might be a good introduction to the parts of the reproductive system of both the male and female, as well as the beginning of an understanding of the vast effects of the action of the pituitary gland.

Text and Library Books:

Burnett, R.W., J.W. Clemensen and H.S. Heyman. *Life Goes On,* second edition. N.Y.: Harcourt, Brace, and World, 1959. (The glossary at the end of this curriculum will provide the teacher with medically accurate definitions and pronunciations for the more difficult words.)
There is also a glossary in the T.A.M.A. Kit No. II: Levin, Adeline L. and Dr. James R. Fox. *Teaching Resource Manual in Human Sexuality Education for Upper Grades.* Minneapolis: *T*eaching *A*ids *M*edically *A*uthenticated, 1968, chapter VIII, pp. 60-67.

Audio-Visual Materials:

Transparencies: "Genitalia—Male" and "Genitalia—Female" from the T.A.M.A. Kit No. II (A-V media kit).
"The Human Reproductive Systems."
Plates: "Female Pelvic Organs," Tampax, Inc. (In classrooms—grade 5.)
"Female Reproductive Organs," Personal Products Company. (In classrooms—grade 5.)
Film: "Girl to Woman," 20 minutes.

3. *Concepts:* The names of the reproductive organs should be clearly understood as well as the precise definition.

Learning Experiences: For each part of the human reproductive system studied, give an accurate definition. This definition should be discussed in class with the teacher so that it is understood. As a result of several problem-solving situations, each student could accumulate and compile his own dictionary of terms. The student would research the initial definitions, but the teacher should examine the final copy and explain any changes made. Throughout the unit encourage youngsters to discuss these concepts with their parents at home. Use and encourage the children to use the correct terminology from this unit in correct context as often as is practical in class discussions so that it becomes a natural part of their vocabulary. When youngsters perform writing activities related to this unit, guide and encourage them to use the correct terminology. At the conclusion of the unit, review the path of the sperm from the testicles to the penis, and the egg cell from the ovary to the uterus, using all the terms from the vocabulary that apply.

Text and Library Books:

Teacher: "From Fiction to Fact." N.Y.: Tampax Corp., 1966, pp. 12-14. (A teaching guide on menstruation and menstrual health—in classrooms—grade 5.)

Ingraham, Hollis S. "The Gift of Life." N.Y.: Health Education Service, State Department of Health, P.O. Box 7283, Albany, N.Y. 12224, 1951.

Pupil: Bauer, W.W. *et al. About Yourself.* Glenview, Ill.: Scott, Foresman and Co., 1962, pp. 273-279.

Hofstein and Bauer. *The Human Story,* pp. 45-46.

Strain, Frances. *Being Born.* N.Y.: Appleton-Century, 1954, pp. 128-134.

Audio-Visual Materials:

Transparencies (with overlay): "Anatomy and Physiology of the Reproductive System—Male" and "Anatomy and Physiology of the Reproductive System—Female" (from T.A.M.A. Kit mentioned previously—A-V media kit).

Transparencies: "The Human Reproductive System."

4. *Concepts:* The testicles affect the growth of boys.

Learning Experiences: Compare a boy in this grade with an older brother in terms of voice, widened shoulder proportion, facial, pubic, and axillary hair.

Text and Library Books:

Hofstein and Bauer. *The Human Story,* pp. 10-15.

Lerrigo, Marion and Helen Southard. "Finding Yourself." Chicago: American Medical Association, 1961, pp. 14-15.

5. *Concepts:* The ovaries affect the growth of girls.

Learning Experiences: Compare a girl in this grade with her older sister in terms of voice, body proportions (rounded hips, fuller breasts), public and axillary hair, and the reasons for each of these developments. Discuss the role of deodorants in preventing unpleasant odors. This should be related to increased perspiration and the different character of perspiration occurring with physical and emotional maturation.

Text and Library Books:

Teacher: "From Fiction to Fact" (Tampax, Inc.), pp. 12-17.

Hofstein and Bauer. *The Human Story,* p. 10.

Lerrigo, Marion and M.A. Cassidy. *A Doctor Talks to Nine to Twelve Year Olds.* Chicago: Budlong Press, 1965, pp. 55-60, 63-66.

Lerrigo and Southard. "Facts Aren't Enough." p. 23.

―――――. "Finding Yourself." pp. 14-15.

Wilcox, Charlotte, and William Boulton. *Stay Healthy.* Chicago: Benefic Press, 1962, pp. 127-156.

6. *Concepts:* Each of the female reproductive organs is designed to perform a definite purpose or task.

Learning Experiences: Provide an explanation of the function of each of the organs in the outline, showing how its design and position enables it to perform its purpose. With a transparency showing the uterus, point out the thick lining of the uterus and how this is good for the growth of the embryo and fetus. Discuss the topic of the sources for our information, having the students compare the information given by their peers with that of parents, teachers, and counselors, pointing out that the latter has more accurate information and more sound advice than the peers. During class discussions care should be taken to see that youngsters understand that all the opinions expressed are not necessarily factual, and should not be taken as correct information. (When wrong information is given in class discussions, the teacher could ask, "Do you all agree?" or "Does someone care to comment?") Hold unhurried question-and-answer periods to discuss questions arising from films, books, etc. Some questions may seem trivial to adults, but they may bother youngsters. Written questions in a question box has proved to be very effective activity for clarifying the different ideas youngsters may have.

Text and Library Books:

Glemser, Bernard. *All About the Human Body.* N.Y.: Random House, 1958, pp. 123-132.

Gruenberg, Sidonie Matsner. *The Wonderful Story of How You Were Born.* Garden City, N.Y.: Doubleday and Company, 1959.

Hofstein and Bauer. *The Human Story,* pp. 16-17, 46.

Lerrigo and Cassidy. *A Doctor Talks to Nine to Twelve Year Olds,* p.17.

Strain. *Being Born.* N.Y.: Appleton-Century, 1954, pp. 6, 11, 134.

Audio-Visual Materials:

Transparencies: "Conception, Prenatal Development and Birth." "The Human Reproductive System."

Plate: Dickinson, Belskie, *Birth Atlas.* N.Y.: Maternity Center Association, Plate 3.

7. *Concepts:* Each of the male reproductive organs is designed to perform a definite purpose or task.

Learning Experiences: Provide an explanation of the function of each of the organs in the outline, showing how its design and position enables it to perform its purpose. If there has not been an opportunity before this to create a question box for the room, a good time to organize one might be after the showing of "Human Growth," since this film provides an opportunity for questioning.

Text and Library Books:

Strain, Frances B. *Being Born.* N.Y.: Appleton-Century, 1954, pp. 7, 23.

Audio-Visual Materials:

Transparencies: "Conception, Prenatal Development and Birth."
Film: "Human Growth," 22 minutes.
Plates: "Female Pelvic Organs" (Tampax, Inc.).
"Female Reproductive Organs" (Personal Products Co.).

8. *Concepts:* Menstruation is a normal, healthy process of the female reproductive system.

Learning Experiences: Discuss the ages when menstrual periods usually begin, the frequency and duration, and how these may vary from girl to girl. Discuss the proper protection and personal cleanliness necessary during the period and how this might be carried out. Discuss the fact that male teachers are aware of these events, understand the young girls' needs, and will be considerate. The film "Boy to Man" could be shown at this time as a review of the unit, as a review of the structure and function of the male and female reproductive systems, and as a help for all to understand male sexual development.

Text and Library Books:

Teacher and Parent: (booklet) "How Shall I Tell My Daughter?" Personal Products Co., Milltown, N.J.
Teacher: (leaflet) Dodge, Eva F. "The Doctor Talks About Menstruation." N.Y.: Tampax, Inc. (reprint), 1966.

Audio-Visual Materials:

Transparencies: "Conception, Prenatal Development and Birth." "The Human Reproductive System."

9. *Concepts:* Sperm cells may be passed from the body during nocturnal emissions, masturbation, or mating. Nocturnal emissions are a normal process of the male reproductive system.

Learning Experiences: After the showing of "Boy to Man," the teacher may wish to probe for questions regarding different aspects of the film. The subject of nocturnal emissions should be looked into far enough to be reasonably sure that the youngsters understand what these emissions are, and that they are a normal process. After the initial probe, if nothing more is asked, the subject could be reviewed quickly by summarizing the positive aspects of Strain's comment *(Being Born,* p. 27) that when it occurs, it is merely evidence that they are growing up, and for this reason they should be proud when it occurs. If further interest is not shown, they could be casually reminded of their opportunity to use the question box before going to the next subject.

Text and Library Books:

Teacher: "From Fiction to Fact" (Tampax, Inc.), pp. 12-17.
Strain, Frances B. *Being Born.* N.Y.: Appleton-Century, 1954, pp. 25-27.

Audio-Visual Materials:

Film: "Boy to Man," 16 minutes.

10. *Concepts:* The youngster may understand much more than before, but is not yet to be a teacher of those who are younger than he.

Learning Experiences: Through classroom discussion it could be illustrated that much like mathematics, where youngsters in kindergarten, grades 1 and 2 are not ready for the concepts of division, neither are they ready for the ideas the fifth graders have just learned.

11. *Concepts:* Preparations need to be made for new babies.

Learning Experiences: Have a youngster whose family has recently had or is about to have a baby report to the class on the preparations that were made.

Text and Library Books:

Lerrigo and Cassidy. *A Doctor Talks to Nine to Twelve Year Olds,* pp. 37-39.
Lerrigo and Southard. "A Story About You," pp. 16-17.

12. *Concepts:* Human reproduction is a miraculous but precise chain of events.

Learning Experiences: In a classroom discussion bring out the miraculous aspects of how two individual cells can contain all the characteristics of heredity and by meeting each other can produce the beginnings of a human life.

Text and Library Books:

Lerrigo and Southard. "A Story About You," pp. 10-11.
Strain, Frances. *Being Born.* N.Y.: Appleton Century, 1954, pp. 42-43.

Audio-Visual Materials:

Sound Color Filmstrip: "Life Begins: Human Reproduction."

13. *Concepts:* Cells are the building blocks of living things.

Learning Experiences: Let students view various kinds of cells through the microscope and afterwards draw diagrams of these cells, create replicas from construction paper, or develop clay models to illustrate cell structures. Brief descriptions of cell functions might then be given.

Text and Library Books:

Burnett, R.W., J.W. Clemensen and H.S. Hoyman. *Life Goes On,* second edition. N.Y.: Harcourt, Brace and World, 1959.
Hofstein and Bauer. *The Human Story,* p. 26.

Audio-Visual Materials:

Slides: "Family Life and Sex Education."

14. *Concepts:* Millions of sperm are produced in the testes.

Learning Experiences: Point out that sperm are cells of human reproduction.

Text and Library Books:

Ingraham. "The Gift of Life."
Smith, Herbert, *et al. Science 6.* River Forest, Ill.: Laidlaw Brothers, 1966, pp. 26-31.

15. *Concepts:* Ova are produced in the ovaries.

Learning Experiences: Hold a classroom discussion on why so many sperm are produced in the male, while only one ovum is produced in the female. Point out that ova are cells of human reproduction.

Text and Library Books:

Farnsworth, Dana. *Choosing Your Goals.* Chicago: Lyons and Carnahan, 1965, p. 196.
Hofstein and Bauer. *The Human Story,* pp. 18-19, 25.
Lerrigo and Cassidy. *A Doctor Talks to Nine to Twelve Year Olds.* pp. 8, 9.

Lerrigo and Southard. "Finding Yourself," pp. 16-17, 22-23.
─────────. "A Story About You," pp. 12-13.
Strain. *Being Born.* N.Y.: Appleton-Century, 1954, pp. 4, 6, 7, 11, 23.

Audio-Visual Materials:

Transparencies: "Conception, Prenatal Development and Birth." "The Human Reproductive System."

16. *Concepts:* There is a definite path that the sperm follow to reach the ovum.

Learning Experiences: Use one of the transparencies listed, or make a diagrammatic blackboard sketch to trace the path of the sperm to the Fallopian tube.

Text and Library Books:

Lerrigo and Cassidy. *A Doctor Talks to Nine to Twelve Year Olds,* pp. 18-22.
Lerrigo and Southard. "Finding Yourself," pp. 17, 21-22, 26.
Weart, Edith. *The Story of Your Glands.* N.Y.: Coward-McCann, Inc., 1963, pp. 15-20, 21-23, 39-46, 52-57, 67, 68.

17. *Concepts:* When the sperm enters the ovum, the miracle of life begins.

Learning Experiences: In a classroom discussion, get the pupils to project the implications behind the fact that only one sperm is allowed to fertilize an ovum.

Text and Library Books:

Hofstein and Bauer. *The Human Story,* pp. 27-28.
Lerrigo and Southard. "Finding Yourself," p. 26.
Strain. *Being Born.* N.Y.: Appleton-Century, 1954, p. 31.

Audio-Visual Materials:

Transparencies: "Conception, Prenatal Development and Birth." "Egg Fertilization and Cell Division," T.A.M.A. Kit No. II (Human Sexuality Education, Upper Grades). "The Human Reproductive Systems."

18. *Concepts:* The new life begins to grow on the lining of the uterus.

Learning Experiences: With a diagram or transparency of the uterus, point out how the fertilized ovum would easily implant itself in the soft, prepared lining of the uterus. (A youngster could be asked to come to the board and draw the uterus on which the explanation and additions would later be made.)

Text and Library Books:

Farnsworth. *Choosing Your Goals,* p. 196.
Hofstein and Bauer. *The Human Story,* p. 28.
Lerrigo and Southard. "Finding Yourself," pp. 26-28.
_____."A Story About You," pp. 17-18.

Audio-Visual Materials:

Transparencies: "Conception, Prenatal Development and Birth."
"The Human Reproductive Systems."

19. *Concepts:* The placenta and umbilical cord are an intricate life-giving network for the embryo.

Learning Experiences: With the aid of the special transparency on the embryo, explain the way in which the egg imbeds itself into the lining of the uterus and the early development of the umbilical cord.

Text and Library Books:

Farnsworth. *Choosing Your Goals,* pp. 192-195.

Audio-Visual Materials:

Transparency: (special) "Conception, Prenatal Development and Birth," (Transparency G with just the two end illustrations showing).

20. *Concepts:* All parts of the body grow and develop in the fetus until it is a complete human being.

Learning Experiences: Have children construct a time line of the development of a given system of the fetus; one group taking the nervous system, another the circulatory system, another the appendages, etc.

Text and Library Books:

Hofstein and Bauer. *The Human Story,* p. 32.
Lerrigo and Cassidy. *A Doctor Talks to Nine to Twelve Year Olds,* pp. 23-31.
Strain. *Being Born.* N.Y.: Appleton-Century, 1954, p. 38.

Audio-Visual Materials:

Illustration: Meilach, Dona and Elias Mandel. *A Doctor Talks to Five to Eight Year Olds.* Chicago: Budlong Press, 1966, p. 43.
Transparencies: "Conception, Prenatal Development and Birth." "How Life Begins."

21. *Concepts:* After nine months of developing the baby is ready to be born.

Text and Library Books:

Hofstein and Bauer. *The Human Story,* p. 34.
Lerrigo and Southard. "A Story About You," pp. 21-23.
Strain. *Being Born.* N.Y.: Appleton-Century, 1954, pp. 54-63.

Audio-Visual Materials:

Transparent Overlay Booklet: "How the Human Baby Grows Inside Its Mother," T.A.M.A. Kit No. II (A-V media kit).
Plates: "Life Before Birth" (*Life* Magazine Series).
Film: "Human Reproduction," 16 minutes.

22. *Concepts:* Birth is a normal process.

Learning Experiences: With the *Birth Atlas* (Dickinson) trace the steps of human birth. Using the *Birth Atlas* and supplemented with their own charts, time lines, etc., have groups of students report on the complete process of birth as a culminating review activity. The teacher may wish to make a point of mentioning that all births do not follow the same procedure. There are such procedures as Caesarean births. Arrange for an unhurried question-and-answer period regularly throughout the term of this unit, so that children may overcome embarrassment and be sure their ideas are correct. (These sessions also help the teacher evaluate attitudes.)

Text and Library Books:

Gruenberg, Sidonie. *The Wonderful Story of How You Were Born.*
Hofstein and Bauer. *The Human Story,* pp. 35-37.
Lerrigo and Cassidy. *A Doctor Talks to Nine to Twelve Year Olds,*
     pp. 32-35.
Lerrigo and Southard. "Finding Yourself," p. 29.
Strain. *Being Born.* N.Y.: Appleton-Century, 1954, pp. 64-84.
Teacher: Burnett, *et al. Life Goes On,* second edition, p. 32.

Audio-Visual Materials:

Plates: Dickinson, Belskie. *Birth Atlas.*
Slide: Meilach and Mandel. *A Doctor Talks to Five to Eight Year
     Olds,* p. 53.
Transparencies: "Conception, Prenatal Development and Birth."

23. *Concepts:* Heredity makes us like our parents.

Learning Experiences: Have class members bring in family portraits, family reunion pictures, and note the similar characteristics. Have each class member construct a family tree listing all the ancestors known. Let each student construct a chart showing the color of eyes of all his ancestors for which this is known. Another chart could be made for hair or other easily identifiable characteristics.

Text and Library Books:

Ames, Gerald and Rose Wyler. *The Giant Golden Book of
     Biology.* N.Y.: Golden Press, 1961, pp. 55-63.
Farnsworth. *Choosing Your Goals,* pp. 198-205.
Glemser, Bernard, *All About the Human Body.* N.Y.: Random
     House, 1958, pp. 123-132.
Hofstein and Bauer. *The Human Story,* pp. 38-41.
Lerrigo and Cassidy. *A Doctor Talks to Nine to Twelve Year Olds,*
     pp. 9-14.
Lerrigo and Southard. "Finding Yourself," pp. 30-31.
_____."A Story About You," p. 27.
Strain. *Being Born.* N.Y.: Appleton-Century, 1954, pp. 105-116.

Audio-Visual Materials:

Film: "Human Heredity," 20 minutes.
Sound Color Filmstrip: "Life Begins: Human Reproduction."

24. *Concepts:* Promiscuity may lead to unwanted children.

Learning Experiences: In a class discussion emphasize the preparations that should be made for a new baby, noting the love of the parents for each other as well as for the coming child and the provisions for physical facilities (bed, shelter, sterilization equipment). The teacher should review the rules of modesty (such as girls' sitting position, mode of dress, etc.) as it relates to molestation and promiscuity. This could be reviewed when discussing proper clothes to wear to school, etc.

Text and Library Books:

Hofstein and Bauer. *The Human Story,* p. 28.
Lerrigo and Southard. "Finding Yourself," pp. 45-46.

Audio-Visual Materials:

Transparencies: "The Human Reproductive Systems."[3]

---

[3] *Guide for Teaching Health in the Area of Human Relations and Sexuality, K-6, 8 and 11.*

CHAPTER 8   *The Curriculum for the Junior Grades*

Levels of Psychosexual Development

The Fourteen- to Sixteen-Year-Old

The fourteen- to sixteen-year-old is essentially self-conscious and self-concerned. He struggles to cope with a changing body image, to develop controls over emotional drives that are more imperative now than they have been at any time since early childhood, and to find a place in the world as an autonomous, decision-making member of society.

At this age one notes a considerable range of physical development. Some may still be at the preadolescent stage; others may have already achieved the physical growth of adulthood. The highest percentage of concerns voiced by youngsters of this age are those that involve physical appearance. Worries about weight, skin problems, and good looks reflect preoccupation with changing bodies. These anxieties are accompanied by fear that all may not turn out well.

Another aspect of this self-consciousness is an easy vulnerability to hurt feelings. Self-esteem is shaky. The testing ground selected for proof of worth is most frequently the area of heterosexual attractiveness. Many young people worry about popularity. Some youngsters withdraw socially so as to protect themselves from rejection. The need is to be accepted, to be attached, to be sought after. Regardless of the facts of their social situation, they are rarely secure in their acceptance by peers and adults. Loneliness is frequently referred to as a problem, particularly by girls. They are looking inward with the question, "Do I have what it takes?"

The questioning of self is accompanied by questioning of the basic assumptions previously taken for granted. They are scrutinizing their religious beliefs and practices. They seek people, especially peers, who demonstrate loyalty, truthfulness, and consistency.

At this stage, attachments to both parents are especially intense and may be full of conflict. On one side of the conflict is renewed possessiveness and demand; on the other, the continued effort to withdraw from dependency. The anxiety that this struggle produces is not far from the surface of the average boy and girl of this age.

One of the ways that family issues are dealt with is to focus on patterns of adulthood. Girls are interested in the roles of womanhood; boys try out the ways of the men who they respect. They shift back and forth from protesting adult ways to assuming such ways themselves. Thus, they become fortified by identifying with both sides of the generation gap.

They are beginning now to test out heterosexual closeness on a more mature level rather than one that primarily meets needs for dependency and attachment. In their hurry, however, they are often pushed to assume precocious postures. The teacher must bear in mind that at this time the youngsters themselves often are aware that they are not yet ready for the behavioral patterns they are assuming. The fact that they are not emotionally ready usually precludes their experiencing pleasure from behavior that is gratifying to those who are more mature. The question arises then as to why youngsters assume such joyless burdens. They do so for various reasons, for example, to meet what they perceive to be the expectations of their peers, to declare to themselves and to the world emancipation from childhood dependence and restrictions, and to provide themselves with practice for the adult patterns that later will be legitimately theirs. Also, one should not underestimate the attraction of risk and limit testing.

It is at this stage and at the next one that their greater comfort and ease with members of the same sex, in combination with unstable controls over sexuality and a quest for adventure, sometimes results in homosexual experimentation, especially on the part of boys. Despite whatever bravura, almost every boy and girl is deeply troubled about being "queer." Homosexual fantasies and homosexual behavior observed in others are as much a source of anxiety as are the firsthand experiences of some adolescents. Almost all of the young people, however, go on to normal heterosexual adjustments in adulthood.

In summary, the teacher of the fourteen- to sixteen-year-old deals with a youngster who is shifting from making excessive demands on adults to protesting even casual interest in his affairs by the same adults. The teacher is dealing with a youngster who is troubled about his acceptability, particularly to peers. He may be struggling in very deep water. Help will come from understanding, acceptance, and from the fortification that results from the knowledge that he is not alone or different in his self-doubts and fears. He is interested in basic physiological information about sexual response, fertilization, and embryology. He is also seriously interested in information about homosexuality, prostitution, venereal disease, abortion, and illegitimacy. He needs to learn how to pace his behavior to his emotional readiness; such readiness will differ widely for children at this age. Practical matters of how to ask for a date, how to act on a date, how to look attractive, and how to be popular are of great interest. Romantic fantasies and reactions to the sexual content of the popular media and to the demands of peers require anchorage. The fourteen- to sixteen-year-old is usually in a stormy phase of adjustment and needs to discuss his questions directly and candidly with informed and understanding adults.[1]

UNIT I: Understanding Adolescent Changes

A. Stages of development
   1. Infancy
   2. Childhood
   3. Adolescence
   4. Adulthood

---

[1] "Family Living Including Sex Education Guide," N.Y.C. Bureau of Curriculum Development, Board of Education, N.Y.C., series 1969-1970.

B. Body structure
   1. Cells
   2. Tissues
   3. Organs
   4. Systems

C. Body and Mind Relationship (Psychosomatic)

D. Importance of Good Mental Health
   1. Behavioral changes
   2. Emotional needs are satisfied differently
   3. Mental disorders
   4. Attitudes toward mental health

E. Endocrine System
   1. Location
   2. Functions
   3. Malfunctions and causes

F. Growth Spurt
   1. Coordination
   2. Susceptibility to disease

G. Secondary Sex Characteristics
   1. Acne
   2. Voice change
   3. Body shape
   4. Genital development and reproduction
   5. Effects on psyche
   6. Energy from new drives

H. New Feelings and Experiences
   1. Menstruation
   2. Seminal emissions
   3. Sex drives
   4. Masturbation[2]

----

[2]*Guide for Teaching Health in the Area of Human Relations and Sexuality K-6, 8 and 11.* Independent School District No. 77, Mankato, Minnesota 56001, 1968. Used by permission.

The Curriculum

Grades 7 and 8

1. *Concepts:* A person passes through different stages of maturity in reaching adult maturity.

Learning Experiences: Discuss what makes one age group completely different from the others regarding habits, growth, and learning experiences.

Text and Library Books:

Diehl, Harold S., *et al. Health and Safety for You,* second edition. N.Y.: McGraw-Hill Book Company, 1964, pp. 15-20.

Audio-Visual Materials:

Film: "Love and the Facts of Life—Growing Up from Childhood to Maturity" No. 2, 16 minutes, 35mm.

2. *Concepts:* Adolescence is a period of development between childhood and adulthood.

Learning Experiences: Write for five minutes on why adolescence is called "The Big Years." In a large group, discuss written comments.

Text and Library Books:

Gallagher, J. Roswell, *et al. Health for Life.* Chicago: Ginn and Company, 1964, pp. 5-18.

3. *Concepts:* Teenagers are people who are between twelve and twenty years of age.

Learning Experiences: Is every adolescent a teenager and vice versa? Is everyone twenty years of age and older an adult?

Text and Library Books:

Peterson, Eleanor M. *Successful Living.* Chicago: Allyn and Bacon, Inc., 1958, pp. 18-19.

4. *Concepts:* Adolescence is a healthy period of life.

Learning Experiences: Why are accidents, homicide and suicide three of the leading causes of teenage deaths? What can be done about them?

Text and Library Books:

Diehl. *Health and Safety for You,* pp. 20-24.

5. *Concepts:* Collections of cells called tissues, organs, and systems form the human body, the most complex structure in existence.

Learning Experiences: Diagram a cell. Studying the function of each part will help in understanding cell division and how the body is developed. Sketch a human body identifying four kinds of tissue, four organs, four systems.

Text and Library Books:

Diehl. *Health and Safety for You,* pp. 28-41.

6. *Concepts:* All body parts are interdependent.

Learning Experiences: Using the circulatory and respiratory systems, explain how the body parts are dependent upon one another.

Text and Library Books:

Diehl. *Health and Safety for You,* pp. 42-47.

7. *Concepts:* The mind is a storehouse of past experiences.

Learning Experiences: Before giving a reading assignment explaining the mind, get the students' oral interpretations of what the mind is. What are the five senses? How are they related to the mind? What are the three parts of the mind?
Explain the importance of the conscious mind, conscience, and unconscious mind. Were you born with a conscience? Where did you get it? Can you destroy or change your conscience?

Text and Library Books:

Gallagher, *Health for Life,* pp. 21-25.

8. *Concepts:* You cannot separate the mind and body.

Learning Experiences: What is meant by the word "psychosomatic"? Give some personal examples showing how the mind affects the body or the body affects the mind.

Text and Library Books:

Diehl. *Health and Safety for You,* pp. 42-44.

Audio-Visual Materials:

Film: "Emotional Health," 20 minutes, 16mm.

9. *Concepts:* Behavior is need satisfaction.

Learning Experiences: Why do we believe the way we do? What are some of the things that influence our behavior?

Text and Library Books:

Diehl. *Health and Safety for You,* pp. 62-72.
Peterson. *Successful Living,* pp. 10-11.

10. *Concepts:* Good mental health results when emotional needs are satisfied.

Learning Experiences: What are the six basic emotional needs that must be satisfied? (*Teacher information:* love, sense of personal worth, achievement, creation, examples in living, and personal philosophy.)

Text and Library Books:

Diehl. *Health and Safety for You,* pp. 50-54.

11. *Concepts:* Emotions are feelings such as love, anger, and fear. Emotional needs are satisfied differently at different age levels.

Learning Experiences: Taking love as an example, how is this emotion satisfied at different age levels? Explain self-love, give-and-take love, romantic love, and altruistic love.

Text and Library Books:

Peterson. *Successful Living,* p. 73.

12. *Concepts:* Emotional needs when satisfied give a person a feeling of security or inner confidence.

Learning Experiences: When watching a person perform a task, how can you tell whether he possesses self-confidence?

Text and Library Books:

Diehl. *Health and Safety for You,* pp. 54-60.

13. *Concepts:* Emotional needs that are not satisfied lead to frustration. Some types of behavior can become a serious problem.

Learning Experiences: When our emotional needs such as achievement are not satisfied, what feelings come to the surface? Are anger and fear always bad? Why or why not? Give personal examples.

Text and Library Books:

Diehl. *Health and Safety for You,* pp. 74.

14. *Concepts:* Immature people do not accept the responsibility for their behavior.

Learning Experiences: Why is the behavior of childhood not acceptable in adolescence? Do you ever exhibit immature behavior? Why? What are regression, rationalization, projection, fantasy, and negativism? Role playing or writing a play are very good ways of helping students remember the use of defense mechanisms.

Text and Library Books:

Diehl. *Health and Safety for You,* pp. 81-84.
Peterson. *Successful Living,* pp. 100-103.

15. *Concepts:* The ability to squarely face yourself indicates maturity.

Learning Experiences: Why must we face our physical and mental capabilities?

16. *Concepts:* Mental illness may be the result if we do not learn to control our emotions and face our problems.

Learning Experiences: What is mental illness? Are we all mentally ill? What causes mental illness?

Text and Library Books:

Diehl. *Health and Safety for You,* pp. 86-100.
Gallagher. *Health for Life,* pp. 381-389.
Peterson. *Successful Living,* pp. 111-116.

17. *Concepts:* Mental illness is quite a common disease.

Learning Experiences: Why is the number of people suffering from mental illness in this country continually increasing?

18. *Concepts:* There are different groups of mental disorders.

Learning Experiences: What are psychoneuroses, psychoses, character disorders, and psychosomatic disorders? Give examples of each.

19. *Concepts:* Most mental illnesses can be successfully treated.

Learning Experiences: Bring in a resource person to talk about causes and prevention of mental illnesses.

20. *Concepts:* Treatment for mental illness may be either psychological or physical.

Learning Experiences: What are some of the methods used in treating the mentally ill? Why are psychodrama and group therapy very successful methods of therapy?

21. *Concepts:* Seek professional help.

Learning Experiences: Who is a quack? List the various professional people involved in psychotherapy. What does each contribute? (Show the film "How Are You?" a second time.)

Audio-Visual Materials:

Film: "How Are You?"

22. *Concepts:* Attitudes toward the mentally ill are changing rapidly.

Learning Experiences: What would be your reaction if a member of your family were to develop a serious mental problem?

23. *Concepts:* Practicing good mental health is the best prevention of mental illness.

Learning Experiences: Write a paragraph on "How I Intend to Maintain Good Mental Health" (ten-minute time limit).

24. *Concepts:* The endocrine system helps to control body growth and body functions by secreting hormones.

Learning Experiences: Locate the endocrine glands on a diagram of the human body. Give the name and function of the hormones each secretes. Examine the effects of improper diet on the endocrine system.

Text and Library Books:

Diehl. *Health and Safety for You,* pp. 356-362.
Gallagher. *Health for Life,* pp. 277-286.
Peterson. *Successful Living,* pp. 26-27.

Audio-Visual Materials:

Film: "Endocrine Glands: How They Affect You," 18 minutes, 16mm, b/w.

25. *Concepts:* Endocrine glands do not always function properly.

Learning Experiences: What conditions develop when the endocrine glands malfunction? How is the diet related to the endocrine system? Reports can be given on such conditions as diabetes, giving symptoms, cures, etc.

26. *Concepts:* The growth spurt does not occur at the same age for all young people.

Learning Experiences: Why aren't all people of the same age the same size? Why are periodic physical examinations especially important during the growth spurt? What does a good physical examination consist of? What does a doctor learn about us in each phase of the examination?

Text and Library Books:

Boyer, Donald Allen. *For Youth to Know.* River Forest, Ill.: Laidlaw Brothers, 1966, pp. 7-15.
Diehl. *Health and Safety for You,* pp. 20-21.
Gallagher. *Health for Life,* pp. 13-18.
Peterson. *Successful Living,* pp. 22-24.

Audio-Visual Materials:

Film: "Your Body During Adolescence," 13 minutes, 16mm, b/w.

27. *Concepts:* Poor muscle coordination may temporarily result from the growth spurt.

Learning Experiences: Have a boy explain why a six-foot-tall eighth grader may not be as good at basketball as his five-foot buddy.

Text and Library Books:

Diehl. *Health and Safety for You,* pp. 39-40.
Gallagher. *Health for Life,* pp. 54-55.

28. *Concepts:* Sore throats are common during the growth spurt.

Learning Experiences: Explain why sore throats are more dangerous than most people think.

Text and Library Books:

Gallagher. *Health for Life,* pp. 186-187.

29. *Concepts:* A sore throat and swollen glands are symptoms.

Learning Experiences: Special reports on such diseases as infectious mononucleosis, rheumatic fever, and strep throat should be given to point out the seriousness of sore throats and swollen glands.

30. *Concepts:* Young people develop secondary sex characteristics.

Learning Experiences: What is acne? What causes the condition at adolescence? What causes the voice to change? Why do mammary glands develop and the female pelvic bone widen? What hormones cause genital development in the male and female? Why does a girl menstruate? Does menstruating have to change her daily habits? What are seminal emissions?

Text and Library Books:

Gallagher. *Health for Life,* pp. 93-94.

31. *Concepts:* Young people are capable of reproduction.

Learning Experiences: Sketch the reproductive and urinary systems. (It is important to show each as a separate system, yet sharing certain parts.) Label the parts and explain the function of each part. *Teacher note:* The films "Boy to Man" and "Girl to Woman" should not be shown unless many in the class did not see the film in the fifth or sixth grades.

Text and Library Books:

Duvall, Evelyn Millis. *Love and the Facts of Life.* N.Y.: Association Press, 1966.
Lerrigo, Marion and Helen Southard. "Facts Aren't Enough." Chicago: American Medical Association, 1962, chapters 1-4.

Audio-Visual Materials:

Transparencies: "Human Reproductive Systems," St. Paul, Minn. *Film:* "The Human Body: The Reproductive System," 13 minutes, 16mm, color.

32. *Concepts:* Childbirths are not all the same.

Learning Experiences: What are the three stages of labor in normal childbirth? What are breech and Caesarean section births?

Text and Library Books:

Johnson, Eric W. *Love and Sex in Plain Language.* N.Y.: J.B. Lippincott, 1967, chapters 2-7.

Audio-Visual Materials:

Films: "Boy to Man," 16 minutes, 16 mm, color.
"Girl to Woman," 16 minutes, 16 mm, color.

33. *Concepts:* Physical changes may cause psychological problems.

Learning Experiences: Explain why physical changes may cause psychological problems. Students should come up with such ideas as: they were not told what to expect during the changes, self-consciousness, and even guilt.

Audio-Visual Materials:

Film: "Love and the Facts of Life—Having a Baby: the Miracle of Creation," No. 3, 18 minutes, 35mm, color.

34. *Concepts:* Energy from new drives and emotions needs to be released.

Learning Experiences: Discuss how young people cope with new feelings resulting from menstruation, seminal emissions, and sex drives. An explanation of masturbation and its effects may be necessary. What is sublimation?

Text and Library Books:

Davis, M. *Sex and the Adolescent.* N.Y.: Dial Press, 1958, chapters 4, 5, 11, 12.

Audio-Visual Materials:

Transparencies: "Factors Influencing the Sex Drive," 3M Company, St. Paul, Minnesota, 1967.[3]

---

[3]*Guide for Teaching Health in the Area of Human Relations and Sexuality K-6, 8 and 11.*

UNIT II. Young People's Problems in Society

A. Basic groups of society
   1. Family
   2. Friends
   3. Church
   4. School
   5. Government

B. Family Problems
   1. Communication
   2. Responsibilities
   3. Privileges
   4. Independence

C. Peers
   1. Conformity or individuality
      a. Grooming
      b. Cheating, stealing, etc.
   2. Parental approval
   3. Difference between friends and acquaintances
   4. Error in judgment

D. Education
   1. Why
   2. When it begins and ends
   3. What kind
      a. Formal or informal
      b. College or vocational-technical
      c. Special
   4. Should increase intelligence
      a. Types of intelligence
         (1) Abstract
         (2) Concrete
         (3) Social
         (4) Special aptitudes

E. Dating
   1. Reasons for dating
      a. It is natural
      b. Affection

      c. Security

      d. Fun

2. Guides to determine dating age

      a. Physical and emotional maturity

      b. Religious belief

      c. Family pattern

      d. Money available

      e. School work and activities

3. General qualities of a good date

      a. Grooming

      b. Poise

      c. Good conversationalist

      d. Common interests and hobbies

      e. Cheerful, positive attitude

      f. Concern for others

4. Kinds of dates

      a. Meeting at social functions

      b. Dutch treat

      c. Boy ask girl

      d. Girl ask boy

      e. Blind date

5. Opportunities for dating

      a. School activities

      b. "Y" activities

      c. Church functions

      d. Home parties

      e. Informal activities

      f. Movies and plays

6. How to get a date

      a. Talking as a group

      b. Telephone

      c. Notes

      d. Direct conversation

      e. Blind date

7. How to refuse a date

      a. When not wanting to date the person

      b. When wanting the date, but busy

      c. Because parents disapprove

      d. Because of illness

8. Dating responsibilities
   a. Inform date as to the nature of the date
   b. Groomed properly
   c. Be on time for and after date
   d. Proper introductions
   e. Indicate amount of money to be spent
9. Problems of dating
   a. Inferiority complex
   b. How often
   c. Steady (advantages—disadvantages)
   d. Kissing
   e. Unwanted advances (petting)
   f. Intercourse
   g. Blind dates
   h. Pick-up dates
   i. Secret dating
   j. Drinking and smoking
   k. Who sets the pattern of behavior
   l. Money
   m. Transportation
   n. Religion
   o. Color or race
   p. How to break up

F. Religion or Philosophy of Life
   1. Importance
   2. Rebellion
   3. Questioning

G. Alcohol, Narcotics, and Tobacco
   1. History
   2. Kinds
   3. Production
   4. Why or why not used
   5. Results from misuse
      a. Social and economic problem
      b. Accidents
      c. Crime
      d. Health damage
      e. Diseases
      f. Affected personality and appearance

6. Everyone has a decision to make

H. Premarital Physical Sex
   1. Mental
      a. Guilt
      b. Loss of self-respect
      c. Anxiety
      d. Psychosomatic illness
      e. Reputation
   2. Pregnancy
      a. Review of reproductive system
      b. Conception
      c. Miscarriage or abortion
   3. Unwed parents
      a. What to do with baby
         (1) Adoption
         (2) Foster home
         (3) Keep
      b. Economic problems
      c. How to return to normal living
   4. Forced marriages
   5. How to prevent pregnancy
      a. Abstinence
      b. Contraceptives

I. Venereal Diseases
   1. Gonorrhea
      (a) Causative agent
      (b) How it spreads
      (c) Incubation period
      (d) Symptoms
      (e) What to do if contracted
      (f) Diagnostic tests
      (g) Treatment
      (h) Dangers to body if not treated
      (i) No immunity
      (j) Epidemiology
      (k) Prevention

   2. Syphilis
      (a) Kinds (active-latent-congenital)
      (b) Causative agent

(c) How it spreads
(d) Incubation period
(e) Symptoms of different stages
(f) What to do if contracted
(g) Diagnostic tests
(h) Treatment
(i) Dangers to body if not treated
(j) No immunity
(k) Epidemiology
(l) Prevention[4]

---

[4]*Guide for Teaching Health in the Area of Human Relations and Sexuality K-6, 8 and 11.*

The Curriculum (continued)

Grades 7 and 8

1. *Concepts:* Societies are basic groups of people.

Learning Experiences: To get the student's ideas of society, have groups of four or five students construct a poster or montage approximately 3' x 4'. The only instructions should be, "Put on the poster what you think society is and your problems in society." When the posters are completed, each group should interpret its own. *Teacher note:* Be sure students understand that in our society some of the basic groups are family, church, school, government, and friends. This work should be done in class over three or four class periods. Using a tape recorder and taking flash pictures add life to the classes.

2. *Concepts:* The family is the cornerstone of society.

Learning Experiences: "Without families the world would crumble." Explain. What is the purpose of the family?

Text and Library Books:

Anderson, Wayne J. *Design for Family Living.* Minneapolis: T.S. Denison and Co., Inc., 1965, pp. 29-30, 363.

3. *Concepts:* Good communication solves many problems.

Learning Experiences: Discuss how poor communication among members of the family causes unnecessary problems.

Text and Library Books:

Gallagher, J. Roswell, *et al. Health for Life.* Chicago: Ginn and Company, 1964, pp. 466-477.
Peterson, Eleanor M. *Successful Living.* Chicago: Allyn and Bacon, Inc., 1958, pp. 228-241.

Audio-Visual Materials:

Films: "The Tuned Out Generation, Part I," 14 minutes, 35mm, color.
"The Tuned Out Generation, Part II," 14 minutes, 35mm, color.

4. *Concepts:* Personal independence is gained and maintained by properly accepting responsibilities and privileges.

Learning Experiences: Make a list of the responsibilities you have in your home. Why do you have these responsibilities? Make a list of responsibilities you could accept to make your home a better cooperative.

Text and Library Books:

Diehl, H.S., *et al. Health and Safety for You,* second edition. N.Y.: McGraw-Hill Book Company, 1964, pp. 130-139.
Duvall, Evelyn Millis. *Love and the Facts of Life.* N.Y.: Association Press, 1966, pp. 16-17, 117-118.
Landis, Paul H. "Coming of Age: Problems of Teen-Agers." PAP 234. N.Y.: Public Affairs Committee, Inc., 1967, pp. 1-12.

Audio-Visual Materials:

Film: "Young Teens and Family Relationships: Helping at Home," 15 minutes, 35mm, color.

5. *Concepts:* Final independence from your family should be earned.

Learning Experiences: As you look ahead, what things will or should your parents expect of you before they allow you to gain independence? To put the foregoing concepts to practical use a "Be Kind to Your Family Week" is very effective. Ideas such as not to fight with family members, do chores responsibly rather than being told, attempt to organize family discussions, etc. This project should be done without the family being informed. Hold a class discussion at the end of the week to get family responses. Was the project a good learning experience?

Audio-Visual Materials:

Film: "Young Teens and Family Relationships: Learning to Understand Your Parents" 15 minutes, 35mm, color.

6. *Concepts:* Individuality and conformity are necessary for a good society.

Learning Experiences: Explain the relationship of grooming to individuality and conformity. Is it good or bad? Who should decide what good grooming is?

Audio-Visual Materials:

Films: "Values for Teenagers: The Choice Is Yours, Part I (Confusions)," 18 minutes, 35mm, color.
"Values for Teenagers: The Choice Is Yours, Part II (Decisions)," 13½ minutes, 35 mm, color.

7. *Concepts:* Peer pressures are the strongest we experience.

Learning Experiences: Discuss cheating, stealing, etc., in order to be a part of a group or "in." What are other reasons for doing the above? Relate back to need satisfaction. Do friends exert pressure on us to do as they do? Do we have many friends? What is the difference between friends and acquaintances? Should our peers be approved by our parents? Do we ever misjudge people? What are the four common mistakes?

Audio-Visual Materials:

Film: "Popularity Problems of Young Teens: How to Keep and Make Friends," 35 mm, SCFS.

8. *Concepts:* Education is a never-ending process. Knowledge can be gained from education. Some people require special education. There is a difference between mental retardation and mental illness.

Learning Experiences: Questions for thought, which can be put on a worksheet.

1. What is education?
2. When does one's education begin? end?
3. What is the difference between informal and formal education?
4. Should everyone go to college?
5. What are vocation or technical schools?
6. Why do some people require special education? Who are the dependent, trainable, and educable people?

7. Why and how have some people without formal education been successful? Is it more difficult today?

Text and Library Books:

Diehl, *Health and Safety for You,* pp. 110-114, 116-124.
Peterson. *Successful Living,* pp. 168-169.
"A World the Right Size," Medical Services Division, Minneapolis Department of Public Welfare, 1965.

Audio-Visual Materials:

Film: "Introducing the Mentally Retarded," 24 minutes, 16mm.

9. *Concepts:* Intelligence is putting knowledge to use.

Learning Experiences: Are we born with intelligence?

10. *Concepts:* Intelligence is the ability to adapt to a situation. General intelligence can be divided into specific kinds of intelligence. Ability to communicate is important.

Learning Experiences: What are abstract, concrete, and social intelligence? What are special aptitudes? What are some of the ways we communicate with others? How does education improve your ability to communicate? Prepared worksheets based on the outline are helpful to the students. Break the class into groups of four or five, segregating boys and girls. When a worksheet is completed, bring the students together in one big circle.

Text and Library Books:

Peterson. *Successful Living,* pp. 36-40.

11. *Concepts:* There are many reasons for dating.

Learning Experiences: Discuss the reasons why people start dating.

Text and Library Books:

Landis, Paul H. *Your Dating Days.* N.Y.: McGraw-Hill Book Company, 1954, pp. 23-27.

Audio-Visual Materials:

Film: "Love and the Facts of Life—Learning About Sex and Love" No. 1, 17 minutes, 35mm, color.

12. *Concepts:* Everyone does not start dating at the same age.

Learning Experiences: Prepare a guide list that determines the age at which people of your age started to or will start to date.

Text and Library Books:

Anderson. *Design for Family Living,* pp. 67-70.
Gallagher. *Health for Life,* pp. 507-508.
Peterson. *Successful Living,* pp. 243-248.

Audio-Visual Materials:

Filmstrip: "The Human Reproductive Systems."

13. *Concepts:* People whom you date should possess socially acceptable personal qualities.

Learning Experiences: Each person will look for certain qualities in the person he or she will date. What qualities are they looking for? These should be general qualities.

Text and Library Books:

Duvall. *Love and the Facts of Life,* pp. 186-190.
Duvall, E.M. *Today's Teen-Agers.* N.Y.: Association Press, 1962, pp. 105-115.

14. *Concepts:* There are other kinds of dates other than boys asking girls.

Learning Experiences: What kinds of dates have you gone on or will you be going on within the next couple of years?

Text and Library Books:

Duvall. *Love and the Facts of Life,* pp. 174, 200-207, 237.

15. *Concepts:* Our society offers many activities for dating.

Learning Experiences: List activities of schools, churches, Y's, and businesses that offer possible places to take a date. Informal dates such as picnics, swimming, and hiking are inexpensive. List other informal activities that offer dating opportunities.

Text and Library Books:

Duvall, Evelyn Millis, *et al. The Art of Dating.* N.Y.: Association Press, 1967, pp. 8-109.

16. *Concepts:* Dating requires skill.

Learning Experiences: Role play the methods of getting a date using group conversations, telephone calls, note passing, and direct conversation. The boy or girl may accept or refuse the date using proper procedure. The groups may also want to do the above using improper procedures. Dramatize the situation of a young man calling at the home of his date. Have some of the members of the class write a play with *this setting:* a young girl's home. *These characters:* the mother or father of the girl, the girl, and the young gentleman caller. The play should include introductions, a conversation between the parents and the caller resulting from the girl's not being ready, the girl's entry into the room, helping the girl with her coat or sweater, leaving the home, giving an explanation of where they are going and the time of return. The above may be done with either proper or improper methods.

17. *Concepts:* Dating presents problems.

Learning Experiences: Have the class break up into appropriate sized groups to discuss the problems of dating listed in unit outline, which have been put on a worksheet. Each group may explore all the problems or the teacher may allow them to choose a certain one. After the groups have finished their work, bring the class together in a circle or other formation conducive to total class discussion. Have the groups relate their information, then open the class for total discussion.

Text and Library Books:

Boyer, Donald Allen. *For Youth to Know.* River Forest, Ill.: Laidlaw Brothers, 1966, chapter 3.

Johnson, Eric W. *Love and Sex in Plain Language.* N.Y.: J.B. Lippincott, 1967, pp. 59-63.

Lonsoncy, Mary J. and Lawrence J. Lonsoncy. *Sex and the Adolescent.* Notre Dame, Ind.: Ave Maria Press, 1971, chapter 14.

18. *Concepts:* Everyone has a religion or philosophy of life.

Learning Experiences: Discuss what religion is. List some of the different religions. Why is it important to everyone? (*Teacher information:* Be prepared to discuss why some teenagers rebel against religion. Questioning one's religion is good, because it now becomes meaningful.)

Text and Library Books:

Anderson. *Design for Family Living,* pp. 361-362.
Peterson. *Successful Living,* pp. 91-92, 220-221.

19. *Concepts:* The use of alcohol, tobacco, and narcotics dates back to primitive and Biblical times. There are many forms of alcohol, tobacco, and narcotics, and they vary in content and methods of production. People use or refrain from using alcohol, tobacco, and narcotics for various reasons.

Learning Experiences: Show the film "Narcotics—The Inside Story" as an introduction. Have each student write thirty questions, ten on each: alcohol, narcotics, and tobacco. These questions should be ones they really want answered. Divide the class into three groups. Each group can work one or two days on each topic, then rotate to another. After three to six days of research, bring the class together for discussion of their questions. (*Teacher's note:* Check to see that the concepts not covered by the students are brought out through other learning experiences before moving to new material.)

Text and Library Books:

Diehl. *Health and Safety for You,* chapter 12.
Gallagher. *Health for Life,* chapter 29.
Irwin, J.W. "High School Hurdles." Columbus: School and College Service, 1965.

_____."Youth Questions Alcohol." Columbus: School and College Service, 1965.

Vogel, Victor H. and Virginia Vogel. *Facts About Narcotics.* Chicago: Science Research Associates, Inc., 1960.

Audio-Visual Materials:

Films: "Alcohol, Narcotics, and Tobacco" (set of 9), 35mm, color.

"Critical Areas of Health" (set of 3), 35mm, color.

"Drug Abuse" (set of 3), 35mm.

"Narcotics—The Inside Story," 12 minutes, 16mm, color.

20. *Concepts:* Misuse of alcohol, narcotics, and tobacco may cause social and economic problems.

Learning Experiences: Figure the cost of smoking for various families. What are some of the articles students could buy or the amount of money students could save for school or other wants?

Text and Library Books:

Cain, A.H. *Young People and Smoking.* N.Y.: John Day and Company, 1964.

Audio-Visual Materials:

Film: "Tobacco and Alcohol: The $50,000 Habit," 35mm.

21. *Concepts:* Misuse of alcohol, narcotics, and tobacco may result in accidents.

Learning Experiences: Role play a teenage beer party. There should be people who drink and do not drink. Transportation home is involved. After-effects of an auto accident can be brought out. What kinds of accidents result from misuse?

Text and Library Books:

Rice, T.B. *Effects of Alcoholic Drinks, Tobacco, Sedatives, Narcotics.* Evanston, Ill.: Harper and Row, 1962.

Vermes, H. *Helping Youth Avoid Four Great Dangers: Smoking, Drinking, VD, and Narcotics.* N.Y.: Association Press, 1966.

Audio-Visual Materials:

Dangerous Drugs Identification Kit. Winston Products for Education, P.O. Box 12219, San Diego, CA 92112.
Marijuana Awareness Wafer. P.O. Box 12219, San Diego, CA 92112.

22. *Concepts:* Use of alcohol, narcotics and tobacco may affect human behavior.

Learning Experiences: What is the relationship of abusive use of alcohol, tobacco, and narcotics to juvenile delinquency and crime?

Audio-Visual Materials:

Film: "Smoke Anyone?", 11 minutes, 16mm, color.

23. *Concepts:* Bodily processes may be affected by the use of alcohol, narcotics, and tobacco.

Learning Experiences: Teacher note: Special emphasis should be given to marijuana and its dangers.

Audio-Visual Materials:

Films: "Digestion in Our Bodies," 11 minutes, 16mm, color.
"Story of the Blood Stream, Part I," 29 minutes, 16mm, color.

24. *Concepts:* Disease may result from the use of alcohol, narcotics, and tobacco.

Learning Experiences: Special reports could be given on cancer, Buerger's disease, emphysema, coronary heart diseases, alcoholism, and cirrhosis of the liver.

Audio-Visual Materials:

Film: "Respiration," 16 minutes, 16mm, b/w.

25. *Concepts:* The use of alcohol, narcotics, and tobacco may detract from your personality and appearance.

Learning Experiences: The students should know what parts of the body are affected by the use of alcohol, narcotics, and tobacco. A rough sketch of the digestive, respiratory, circulatory systems, and brain can be made. However, the purpose should be mainly to emphasize the location and function of the parts affected.

Audio-Visual Materials:

Film: "Popularity Problems of Young Teens: The Smoking Problem," 35mm, color.

26. *Concepts:* Each individual must decide if he will use tobacco, narcotics, or alcohol.

Learning Experiences: Write a paper explaining why you think you will or will not use alcohol, narcotics, or tobacco. What has influenced you to make these decisions? Your paper is entirely your property and will be held in the strictest confidence. (Ten-minute time limit).

27. *Concepts:* Premarital sex may cause many kinds of problems.

Learning Experiences: Following the viewing of "Sex: A Moral Dilemma for Teenagers," the class can become one large circle for discussion. Parts I and II should be shown on separate days, which will give the students a chance to discuss the remarks they jotted down.

Text and Library Books:

Duvall. *Love and the Facts of Life,* pp. 151-169.
_____. *Today's Teenagers,* pp. 117-131.
Lonsoncy. *Sex and the Adolescent,* chapters 16, 17.
Southard, Helen F. *Sex Before Twenty: New Answers for Young People.* N.Y.: Dutton and Company, 1971.

Audio-Visual Materials:

Films: "Sex: A Moral Dilemma for Teenagers," Part I, 14 minutes, 35mm.
"Sex: A Moral Dilemma for Teenagers," Part II, 20 minutes, 35mm.

28. *Concepts:* Mental problems may result from premarital physical sex.

Learning Experiences: Ask the students to explain how a member of their sex might react mentally after having premarital intercourse. It should be explained by the instructor that this is a hypothetical case; but may become a reality quicker than they think, if they do not think.

Text and Library Books:

Landers, Ann. *Ann Landers Talks to Teen-Agers About Sex.* N.J.: Prentice-Hall, Inc., 1963.

29. *Concepts:* Sexual intercourse sometimes results in an unwanted pregnancy.

Learning Experiences: The instructor must be sure at this time that the student thoroughly understands what causes a pregnancy. An explanation by the teacher of penal erection, what causes the ejaculation of semen, and where the semen is deposited may be necessary.

30. *Concepts:* Young girls sometimes become pregnant.

Learning Experiences: Discuss reasons why some unmarried girls want to become pregnant.

Text and Library Books:

Duvall. *Love and the Facts of Live,* pp. 152-156.
Johnson. *Love and Sex in Plain Language,* pp. 54-57.

31. *Concepts:* Unwed pregnant girls and the young men involved have many decisions to make. Forced marriages lead to more problems.

Learning Experiences: Buzz groups of segregated boys and girls listing what they think their responsibilities would be is effective. Each group should select a recorder so all ideas are reported when the class comes together, in about ten minutes.

32. *Concepts:* Most unwanted pregnancies can be prevented.

Learning Experiences: The instructor should also be able to explain what the various contraceptives are.

Text and Library Books:

Johnson. *Love and Sex in Plain Language,* pp. 47-53.

Audio-Visual Materials:

Film: "Love and the Facts of Life—Contraceptive Methods" No. 5 (Part II), 2 minutes, 35mm, color.

33. *Concepts:* Venereal disease education is imperative.

Learning Experiences: Give each student the junior high pretest from the teaching guide *Venereal Disease Education.* Do not have the students correct the test since it will be given later as a posttest. Each student should be given a programmed learning manual entitled *Facts About Syphilis and Gonorrhea.* The student should work at his own speed, but only in class. The student should not write in the book but record his answers in his notebook along with notes he thinks to be very important. The test in the *Instructor's Handbook* should be given as instructed. If the manual *Facts About Syphilis and Gonorrhea* is not available, have the students research a study sheet in the library or classroom. This sheet should contain a list of vocabulary words pertinent to this topic. Magazine and newspaper articles should be looked up and brought to class to show that V.D. is in an epidemic stage.

Text and Library Books:

Boyer. *For Youth to Know,* pp. 50-56.
Cornacchia, H.J. *Dimensions in Health, Venereal Diseases.* Chicago: Lyons and Carnahan, 1966.
Duvall. *Love and the Facts of Life,* pp. 158-161.
Johnson. *Love and Sex in Plain Language,* pp. 57-59.
Schwartz, W.F. *Facts About Syphilis and Gonorrhea.* Washington, D.C. AAHPER, 1965.
Webster, B.W. *What You Should Know About V.D. and Why.* N.Y.: Scholastic Book Co., 1967.

Audio-Visual Materials:

Film: "A Quarter Million Teenagers," 16 minutes, 16mm, color.

34. *Concepts:* Venereal diseases are communicable.

Learning Experiences: What are some of the ways people have been led to believe that V.D. can be transmitted? Why is V.D. so prevalent among prostitutes and homosexuals?

Audio-Visual Materials:

Film: "Venereal Disease and Your Health," 13 minutes, 35mm, color.

35. *Concepts:* Bodily damage done by V.D. cannot be corrected.

Learning Experiences: Special reports on paresis and congenital syphilis should be given.

Audio-Visual Materials:

Film: "The Innocent Party," 17 minutes, 16mm, color.

36. *Concepts:* V.D. can be prevented.

Learning Experiences: Why is it important to go to a physician for treatment of V.D.?

37. *Concepts:* Venereal diseases could be eradicated.

Learning Experiences: Give the pretest as a posttest. Have the students correct this test and the one given at the beginning of the unit. Allow the students to make a comparison of their tests. Be sure each student understands why he missed any questions on the last test. To check for proper attitudes regarding venereal diseases, give the Attitude-Opinion from *Venereal Disease Education.* If a student gets a question wrong, have him explain his answer, then try to help him acquire the most acceptable attitude.

38. *Concepts:* Young people's problems must be coped with.

Learning Experiences: We have studied subjects you indicated are problems to people of your age. Do you now feel you are capable of making more mature decisions regarding these problems? What particular problems still seem unanswered?

Text and Library Books:

Johnson. *Love and Sex in Plain Language,* chapter 13.
Peterson. *Successful Living,* chapter 32.

39. *Concepts:* Complete maturity is a goal. To reach maturity one must know oneself.

Learning Experiences: Does maturity today mean maturity three years from now? One or two class periods should now be allowed for students to write a confidential paper based on "Who Am I?" "What Is My Purpose?" "This Is What I Believe," or "Where Have I Been and Where Do I Go from Here?" (Any information in these papers must not be passed on without the consent of the student.) Remarks such as, "This is completely wrong," should not be written on the paper. If there is something that you think warrants reconsideration, something as, "Have you thoroughly thought about this?" could be written on the paper or discussed with the student.

Audio-Visual Materials:

Film: "Love and the Facts of Life—Who Am I?" No. 5, 11 minutes, 35mm, color.[5]

---

[5] *Guide for Teaching Health in the Area of Human Relations and Sexuality, K-6, 8 and 11.*

CHAPTER 9   *How to Vary the Sex Education Curriculum to Meet the Needs of Individual Students and Parents*

After your curriculum committee has carefully reviewed chapters 5 through 8, it may be decided changes should be made. The following scope and sequence may also be considered.

Scope and Sequence

The scope and sequence contains generalizations to be developed in the broad area of family living, which includes sex education. It is understood that this scope and sequence is flexible and may be adapted to meet the needs of children at different maturity levels and shaped by the many factors that influence children in a large urban community.

For selected aspects of this curriculum, separate classes for boys and girls may be desirable. If classes are separated, the same content should be taught to both boys and girls.

Prekindergarten—Grade Two

A man and a woman who love each other marry and form a new family.

189

Each member of the family is important as an individual and
  as a member of the family group.
Members of a family do things to help one another.
Curiosity about oneself and others is natural.
Girls grow into women, and boys grow into men.
Living things produce other living things of the same kind.
Human beings and most other animals begin their lives as
  eggs.
There is a growth process before birth.
Parents prepare for the birth of offspring.
Babies need love, time, and care in order to grow and
  develop.

Grade Three—Grade Four

Parents vary in the amount of care they give their offspring.
Successful family living requires sharing for the common
  good.
Men and women have overlapping roles in the home and in
  the world of work.
Children of the same family may be alike in some ways and
  different in other ways.
Friendship involves a special kind of feeling toward another
  person.
* Some animal eggs are fertilized outside the mother's body,
  some inside. Some fertilized eggs grow into babies inside
  the mother's body, some outside.
* An egg from the mother and a sperm from the father unite to
  produce a fertilized egg that grows into a baby.
* Fertilized eggs vary in the time needed to produce a new
  individual.
* Animals and human beings vary in the number of offspring
  produced at a given time.

Grade Five—Grade Six

Each member of the family is entitled to respect and
  reasonable privacy.

---

*Items with asterisks are expanded upon in the next section.

Many forces influence the individual's social behavior.

Boys and girls need a variety of social and recreational activities.

Men and women have overlapping social vocational roles.

Heredity is a factor that influences growth and development.

Environment is a factor that affects physical growth and development.

Nutritional needs during preadolescence require special attention.

Many changes occur at the preadolescent period.

* Puberty initiates physical changes leading to manhood and womanhood.
* Emotional changes accompany physical changes during preadolescence.
* All living things are made of cells.
* Human babies develop from fertilized eggs.
* Human babies grow and develop during the gestation period.

Grade Seven–Grade Nine

Environmental forces influence family living.

Personal decisions reflect one's values and require that one accept responsibility for their outcomes.

Interpersonal relationships develop through a variety of social activities.

Dating in adolescence may provide a basis for development of more lasting relationships.

Accepting responsibility in boy-girl relationships is related to social and emotional maturity.

Tensions during adolescence may arise from a variety of factors.

The endocrine system influences appearance, body functions, and mental and emotional behavior.

Puberty initiates physical changes leading to manhood and womanhood.

All living things are made of cells.

Human babies develop from fertilized eggs.

Human babies grow and develop during the gestation period.

An individual's physical traits are the product of his heredity.[1]

Please note that in the first curriculum given in chapters 5 through 8 there is care to avoid drawing any similarity between lower forms of life and human beings. In the sample lessons that follow, the latter approach is taken.

These lessons are taken from the short syllabus provided above (grades three and four).

Generalization: *Some animal eggs are fertilized outside the mother's body, some inside.*
Some fertilized eggs grow into babies inside the mother's body, some outside.

Content	Learning Activities
Fish and frog eggs are fertilized externally and grow into babies outside the mother's body.	Show pictures of fish and/or frogs' eggs in water. In the springtime visit a local pond or lake to collect frogs' eggs. Put the eggs into an aquarium with pond water. Have children report daily observations of the development of the eggs. (The teacher emphasizes that the female fish and frog squeeze the eggs into the water. The males squeeze sperm into the water near the eggs. The sperm swim to the eggs and fertilize them. This is external fertilization.) View an appropriate film on fertilization.
Turtle and chicken eggs are fertilized internally but grow into babies outside the mother's body.	Display pictures of turtle and chicken eggs. View film on laying of eggs by turtles and chickens. The

---

[1] "Family Living Including Sex Education Guide," N.Y.C. Bureau of Curriculum Development, Board of Education, New York City, series 1969-1970.

The eggs of gerbils, hamsters, mice, dogs, cats, horses, and elephants are fertilized internally and grow into babies inside the mother's body.

teacher emphasizes that in turtles and chickens the sperm from the male joins the egg inside the mother's body. This is internal fertilization. The egg then moves outside the mother's body and develops.

Visit the nature room in the school, a local pet shop, or zoo to observe that some animals keep their babies inside their bodies until they are ready to be born.

Generalization: *An egg from the mother and a sperm from the father unite to produce a fertilized egg that grows into a baby.*

Content

A mother has two ovaries inside her body. Ripe eggs are produced in the ovaries. The father has two testes outside his body. Ripe sperm are produced in the testes. The union of ripe egg and ripe sperm produces a fertilized egg.

The eggs of human mothers are fertilized internally and develop inside the mother's body.

Learning Activities

Use models or overhead projector and/or chalkboard to show simplified diagrams of female and male reproductive organs. Show diagrams of eggs and sperm. (Explain that these are magnified.) View appropriate films.

Generalization: *Fertilized eggs vary in the time needed to produce a new individual.*

Content

The fertilized eggs of some animals develop for a short time before the baby animal is fully formed and ready to be born.

The fertilized eggs of some animals develop for a long time before the

Learning Activities

Discuss the length of time it takes to hatch a chicken's egg.

Have children research and report how long it takes other fertilized

Content (continued)	Learning Activities (continued)
baby animal is fully formed and ready to be born.	eggs to develop fully.
From fertilized egg to hatching:	Record findings on an information chart using pictures drawn or collected by the children. Note length of development period for each. Include some of the following: insects (housefly, moth), fish (guppies, salmon), amphibians (frogs, toads), reptiles (snake, turtle), birds (chicken, sparrow), mammals (dog, cat, elephant, cow).
Name and Development Time _____ _____ _____ _____ _____ _____ _____	
	Use a calendar to demonstrate the length of the human gestation period.

Generalization: *Animals and human beings vary in the number of offspring produced at a given time.*

Content	Learning Activities
Some animal mothers have many babies at one time.	View films that show the number of offspring produced by fish, frogs and turtles. Have children tell about litters produced by their pets (cats, dogs, white mice).
Some animal mothers have only a few babies at a time.	
Some animal mothers have only one baby at a time.	Visit a local pet shop or zoo to check on the number of offspring of domestic and wild animals. Read books dealing with animal litters.
Human mothers usually have only one baby at a time; some mothers have two or more babies at one time.	
	Have children tell about twins in their own families or families of their friends.
	Invite a mother of twins to school to tell how she cares for two babies at the same time.

The following lessons are from grades 5-6.

Generalization: *Puberty initiates physical changes leading to manhood and womanhood.*

Content	Learning Activities
The major changes that take place at puberty are caused by hormones from the pituitary gland and the sex glands. The sex glands (gonads) are the ovaries in the females and the testes in males. The ovaries begin to release mature eggs. The menstrual cycle starts.	View appropriate films on physical changes occurring during puberty.
Menstruation involves the following: One ripe egg is released from an ovary and moves to a Fallopian tube about once every twenty-eight days. In the meantime the wall of the uterus thickens and becomes full of capillaries. The egg is moved along the Fallopian tube toward the uterus. If the egg is not fertilized, it breaks up and dissolves. After some time, the extra thickness of the wall of the uterus, some blood and fluid leave the body through the vagina. This is called the menstrual flow.	Show film on menstruation. Lead the discussion. Invite the school nurse to discuss further the hygiene of menstruation.
In the testes, sperm begin to develop. At times, semen that has sperm in it is released while the boy is sleeping. This is called a nocturnal emission or wet dream.	Prepare boys for the experience of nocturnal emission. Assure them that this can happen to any boy.
The age when puberty begins varies with individuals. Secondary sex characteristics develop:	Provide opportunities for pupils to submit unsigned questions as a basis for further discussion.

Boys

Body fills out. Shoulders and chest broaden. Beard begins to grow. Hair appears under the arms and in the

Content (continued)	Learning Activities (continued)
Boys (continued) pubic region. Changes occur in the activity of the oil and sweat glands. Voice deepens.	
Girls	
Breasts develop. Body rounds out. Hips broaden. Hair appears under the arms and the pubic region. Changes occur in the activity of the oil and sweat glands.	
Parallel to the physical changes in puberty is the continuing development of sexual feelings. At one stage in the sexual maturity of young people, the practice of masturbation may arise. There is no scientific evidence to indicate that masturbation is harmful, but attitudes toward it vary.	Since attitudes toward masturbation vary, it is suggested that questions about masturbation be referred to the child's parents and/or to experts in the fields of medical, psychological, and clerical guidance.

Generalization: *Emotional changes accompany physical changes during preadolescence.*

Content	Learning Activities
Body changes and growth spurts are a normal part of growing up.	Prepare pupils for emotional changes by showing a film dealing with feelings of inadequacy in the early adolescent.
Feelings of inadequacy are sometimes related to rapid and uneven physical changes.	Invite a guidance counselor to lead a discussion on the problems arising from rapid and uneven physical change.
Accepting one's capabilities and limitations is a factor in achieving and maintaining emotional health.	Have pupils read and discuss stories or biographies of young people who overcame problems of adolescence.
	Assure students that maturing slowly is not a physical disability.

Generalization: *All living things are made of cells.*

Content	Learning Activities
All living things are made of protoplasm, which has a colorless, jelly-like appearance. Protoplasm is organized into tiny packages called cells. Each cell consists of a nucleus and cytoplasm inside of a thin sac called a cell membrane.	Show a diagram of a typical animal cell on a wall chart or on a transparency.
Sperm and eggs are cells. Sperm cells develop in organs called testes, part of the male reproductive system. Egg cells develop in organs called ovaries, part of the female reproductive system.	Display charts and pictures of various types of human cells including sperm and egg cells.
Cells differ in size, shape and function. Groups of cells are organized into tissues (bone, muscle, skin), which have specialized functions.	Use a microscope with prepared slides to show types of human cells and human tissues.
Tissues are organized into organs and organs into systems (circulatory, digestive, skeletal, reproductive, etc.).	View a model of a human torso showing the interrelationships of organs and body systems. Illustrate human male and female reproductive systems through diagrams and/or transparencies.

Generalization: *Human babies develop from fertilized eggs.*

Content	Learning Activities
The joining of an egg cell and a sperm cell is necessary to start a new individual.	View a film on fertilization.
Approximately every twenty-eight days a ripe egg cell leaves an ovary and is moved into an oviduct (Fallopian tube).	Follow on a chart the route of an egg cell from ovary, into the oviduct, uterus, and vagina.
When the sperm cells enter the female, the sperm cells swim from	Indicate the path of sperm cells from testes through the penis.

Content (continued)	Learning Activities (continued)
the vagina along the walls of the uterus into an oviduct (Fallopian tube).	
The union of a sperm cell and an egg cell is called fertilization.	Show a diagram of a sperm cell entering an egg cell, and a fertilized egg attached to the wall of the uterus.
The fertilized egg cell begins to divide and is moved toward the uterus where, as it grows, it embeds itself in the thick, soft lining. A fertilized egg cell grows into a new individual.	

Generalization: *Human babies grow and develop during the gestation period.*

Content	Learning Activities
In the uterus, the embryo develops a spongy disc with many tiny, fingerlike projections (placenta). The fingerlike projections protrude into the wall of the uterus. After eight weeks, the embryo is called a fetus.	Show a diagram and/or a transparency of a human embryo with its umbilical cord and placenta attached to the wall of the uterus.
Between the placenta and the embryo, a long cord (umbilical cord) is developed. The cord contains large blood vessels. In the placenta, food and oxygen pass from the blood of the mother into the blood of the fetus.	
Wastes from the fetus pass through the umbilical cord to the placenta and then into the blood of the mother.	Indicate on a chart the path of wastes from the embryo to the blood of the mother.
The fetus grows and is protected by a liquid and the amniotic sac, which shields it from jars and jolts.	Use diagrams, transparencies, and pictures to show a fetus surrounded by liquid and the amniotic sac.

As the months pass, the mother's uterus keeps stretching to accommodate the growing fetus.

A full-term pregnancy lasts about 280 days or approximately nine months.

When the time comes for the baby to be born, muscles in the uterus begin moving the infant out of the uterus and through the vagina.

Use a series of models showing the birth of a baby.

At the first signs of labor, mothers in this city usually get medical help. Most babies are born head first. Once the delivery is completed, the umbilical cord is tied and severed without causing pain to mother or baby.

The remainder of the cord, the placenta, and the extra thickness of the uterine wall are then expelled (afterbirth).[2]

It is suggested your committee may wish to write to other school districts for additional materials, which might supply ideas for conceptual contents as well as for activities. Some you might find helpful besides those mentioned in the footnotes are:

Parsippany-Troy Hills Township Schools, *Human Sexuality,* Parsippany-Troy Hills Board of Education Curriculum Materials Center, Box 52, Parsippany, N.J. 07054.

Health Education Curriculum Guide, State of Delaware (Department of Public Instruction).

Everything You've Always Wanted to Know About Health Education but Were Afraid to Ask, Anchorage Borough School District, Anchorage, Alaska.

---

[2]"Family Living Including Sex Education Guide."

Health Education K-12—Guidelines for Curriculum Development, Division of Instructional Services, Kansas State Department of Education, Topeka, Kansas.

Determining Other Topics to Include

A survey of the material given in the previous chapters and this one can help your committee to decide which topics you feel are needed by students and parents in your community, and where you would like the greatest emphasis placed.

You may discover that even where it is difficult to institute a full program, partial programs (dealing with subjects such as venereal disease) may be placed in the health education or other existing curricula. Furthermore, such topics as mental health may often be added without any controversy whatsoever.

In connection with venereal disease, we suggest you obtain the booklet "VD," published by McKesson Laboratories, Fairfield, Conn. 06430. It is one your young people will read and remember. It's done in cartoons and a light breezy style, which they find appealing. The vocabulary is such that even slow learners will be able to comprehend it, and the message is one we must get across.

Introducing the Mental Health Aspect

The following topics can be added to any existing health education curriculum.

Mental Health Curriculum for Young Children

Objectives	*Suggested Activities*
To develop self-confidence away from home.	Through assigning room responsibilities make each student feel secure in being an important part of the room.
To develop the belief that one can succeed if he tries.	
To learn to accept failure in its proper perspective.	Talk about how we are different and how we are alike.
To develop a feeling of security.	How would I want others to treat me when this happens to me?
To understand that it is fun to share with others.	Encourage a shy child to first talk

To develop tolerance.
To develop the belief that one can accomplish things and solve problems.
To develop sympathetic attitudes.
To develop a sense of fairness and cooperation.
To develop qualities of leadership and following.

in small groups, then work up to large groups.
Explain only one person or team wins and we must have losers whenever we play games.
To develop tolerance you must have understanding. Help students understand.
Give the timid child opportunity to be chairman of a group activity.
Discussion: Accepted behavior. Respect for other's contribution. Build up self-confidence. Each child should succeed at something each day.
In an art lesson discuss the different types of pictures and find something constructive about each project.
Have a discussion period in which children may discuss failure and success.
Have a number of times for sharing belongings through a planned period.

Curriculum for the Middle Grades

Objectives

Suggested Activities

To understand why a person becomes angry.
To develop the ability for one to stand up for one's rights.
To develop the ability to find pleasure in accomplishments and relationship with others.
To develop a feeling of belongingness.
To develop a respect for another's property.

Do some role playing—make some pictures to emphasize person's feelings.
Think of something that has made you unhappy or angry and what happened or what changed your angry feelings to more pleasant ones.
Give dramatic presentation using open-ended situations about one's rights and one's property. Discuss several endings for each situation. Could use classroom situations that have happened. Work in small

Objectives (continued)   *Suggested Activities (continued)*

groups and let children accomplish some small success in the group.

Have children think of the ways others depend upon them. Help develop a sense of belonging. Class discussion of stories without endings or with several possible endings.

Talks by psychologists. Have students develop lists of courtesy words.

Let children discuss the need for respect for another's property.

Have students develop a bulletin board depicting respect for property—not walking on lawns, etc.

Mental Health for the Intermediate Grades

Objectives   *Suggested Activities*

To develop qualities so as to be accepted by members of own sex.
To develop appropriate behavior toward own peers.
To develop confidence in relationship with adults.
To develop respect for relationship with adults.
To develop confidence in own ability.
To develop feeling of security at home and school.
To develop qualities of honesty, truthfulness and reliability.
To develop sympathy, cooperativeness and interest in others.

Invite a psychiatrist or psychologist to visit class. A guidance counselor could speak on mental health and the development of good relationships with others.

Much more communication among students and adults—group discussions.

School assemblies and good pep assemblies develop school spirit—awards, merits—delegation of authority—letting students earn these through their ability.

Qualities of girl.

Qualities of guy.

What rights do we have, not have.

How can we learn to feel for others?

Are we really interested in others?

Discuss subjects of making friends, popularity, manners and etiquette.
Discuss personality development, adjustment problems and growing toward maturity.
Make a personal list of qualities you admire in someone.
Project students in roles of responsibility.[3]

The Problem of Divorce; Its Effect on the Wife and Husband and on Young Children

The divorce rate among those married in their teens is three to four times higher than that of any other age group. We believe that even in the early years of our children's education this topic should be discussed, particularly if the divorce rate has shown an increase in your community as it has throughout the nation.

We suggest this topic be added to the junior grades curriculum. Possibly the best way in which this can be done is to invite knowledgeable persons—lawyers, members of the clergy, social workers, psychiatrists, psychologists—to form a committee along with educators to work out the special portion of the curriculum dealing with this topic. It should be approached with these basic aspects in mind:

(a) The effect divorce has on children whose parents are divorced. Please point out the large number of divorces among persons you (the teacher) know personally. Some children are ashamed and feel guilty because of their parents' problems. They believe they are the only ones whose parents are splitting up. We have found that the knowledge that other boys and girls are in the same situation is a help to them.

---

[3] "Health Education K-12 Guidelines for Curriculum Development," Division of Instructional Services, State Department of Education, Topeka, Kansas. Prepared by Carl J. Haney, Specialist—Health Education.

(b) The effect divorce has on children whose parents are in the process of divorcing.
(c) The effect divorce has on young people who marry and then divorce.
   1. The effect on the person who wishes to break up the marriage.
   2. The effect on the person who is being divorced.

Hopefully our sex education courses throughout the nation will eventually help to cut down the number of divorces. However, this will not happen unless we accept the fact that many people come into marriage unprepared for it. There are so many young men and women with no idea whatsoever of what marriage entails, who see it as it is portrayed in the television commercials. By including the topic of divorce in our sex education program, perhaps the realities of the situation can be brought to the fore. As the *Washington Post* put it in an editorial of May 31, 1973: "The lack of preparation for marriage often means that when the hard days of sacrifice and responsibility come, the individuals may be taken by surprise. America spends large amounts of time and money preparing our young to be soldiers, workers or whatever, but hardly a thought is given to preparation for parenthood; ironically it is the one career that can be the most demanding and perplexing."

The Role of Counseling in the Sex Education Program

It is our belief that, along with the sex education program, there should be time given to the teachers to work with children on an individual basis. The teacher of sex education must develop a special rapport with his or her students if the program is to be at all effective. This rapport should not be restricted to the classroom; it should be utilized to develop a closer relationship with *each child who needs that relationship.* Not every child does, but there are those who do, who have questions they have to ask and problems they must have answered.

The following note speaks for itself. It was received by a person who had developed rapport with a very troubled eighth grade boy, a fourteen-year-old who had been held over and who was very mature physically for his age.

Will someone help me?

Please help me. I can't take the way I act any more. I yell at my mother and father. And I am going to take drugs to find what's going on inside of me. I just can't stay in one place. What I mean by that is I can't find the good in me. I wish I could love my father and mother. They have a ruff time with me. I yell at them till I get my own way. I just can't stop. I will keep it up till I can't take it. Maybe I am crazz *(note spelling)* like people say I am. I am sad and trying to *(note—word omitted)* myself happy. I wish I could show people I am good but I can't. Maybe God can help me. If there is one. The only one who understands me is Mrs. K. But maybe she don't know me that good. What I mean is that if she knew the way I act at home some times she would not believe it. I tell her what I do at home. But to see it she wouldn't believe it. I think every day I am killing my father yelling at him.

I am a person who can't understand myself. May God forgive for everything. I wrote this then I would have to think about it.

This is not fiction. There is one deletion to protect the child, because the incident to which he refers would reveal his identity.

This child is obviously a very troubled youngster. However, he had attached himself to the author rather than a guidance counselor or social worker because he desperately needed acceptance, although his note reveals how difficult it was for him to accept it.

In the cases of such very troubled children, referral should be made to the guidance counselors and to outside agencies. However, if a child resists, then the educator she (or he) has chosen must be the one to try to help.

That there must be counseling in conjunction with the sex education program is an absolute necessity. Incidentally, we do not mean to imply that the parents should be forgotten in this effort. Far from it. The counselors (be they teachers or professional counselors) should, *after they get the child's permission,* communicate with the parents. They should impress the youngster with the need for involving the parents. Sometimes, however, parents are uncooperative. (In the case of the child who wrote the note, it was extremely difficult to get the parents to see anyone connected with the school. They were in once, refused countless invitations, and have made many appointments and never kept them.) Help should be made available to both young people and adults.

It is important to make known to your teachers of sex education where there is assistance available for young people outside of school, but within the community. Social service agencies and boards of health are two of the major sources.

To cite only one example of why this is necessary, let's look at the statistics in regard to venereal disease. It has been reliably estimated that 3,000 teenagers and young adults are stricken daily. In spite of the fact that penicillin is so very effective in the treatment of V.D., there were 6,251 cases of syphilis reported in 1957, 20,186 cases reported in 1970. There were 216,476 cases of gonorrhea reported in 1957, 573,200 reported in 1970. *And these are only the reported cases.* There are a huge number that go unreported. To turn our backs on this problem is to court disaster. To pay only lip service in the fight against it is ridiculous. To think our children are immune is nonsense. And to think they will always turn to their parents for help is unrealistic.

Parents, too, may need assistance. Referrals to the same agencies may be made. Remember, in dealing with both children and adults confidentiality is extremely important. Nothing can destroy faith more than a revelation of a child's or an adult's problems without his or her consent. We have found that most of the time consent is given after explanations have been made. However, confidences should never be broken, even if it takes hours of work to convince the person of the need to convey the information.

CHAPTER 10

How to Continually
Evaluate the
Sex Education Program

As has been stressed in previous chapters, the sex education program must begin with a series of key objectives. Because of their relationship to evaluation, we should review these goals:

1. To provide the individual with adequate information about his own physical, mental and emotional maturation processes as related to sex.
2. To alleviate fears and anxieties relative to individual sexual development.
3. To develop objective and understanding attitudes toward sex in all of its various manifestations—in the individual, toward himself, and toward others.
4. To give the individual insight concerning his relationships to members of both sexes and to help him understand his obligations and responsibilities to others.
5. To provide enough information about the misuses and deviations of sex to enable the individual to protect himself against exploitation and against injury to his physical and mental health.
6. To provide a climate for learning and the understanding that will enable each individual to utilize his sexuality effectively and creatively in his several roles, i.e., as a child, youth, spouse, parent, community member, and citizen.
7. To build an understanding of the need for and appreciation of moral and ethical values that are necessary to provide a

rational basis for making decisions concerning *all* human behavior.

8. To provide information as to the place of the family in our society and the skills that lead to a responsible home and family life.

9. To provide information and guidance about the emerging social problems that affect the family in our society such as birth control and the population explosion, illegitimacy, early marriage, venereal disease, solo parenthood, divorce, and sexual deviation.

The objectives will enable you to recognize whether or not the program is accomplishing what it set out to accomplish.

Without constant evaluation, this program or any program can easily fall flat. A curriculum is a vital, living thing that must be conveyed to the students. It is not something to be written up in books and then forgotten about or, as so often happens, observed in the breach.

You will need, and hopefully have, the enthusiasm of your faculty. This includes both the teachers involved in actually teaching the course, and the other members of the staff as well. Enthusiasm does a great deal to carry a program at the beginning, but it cannot suffice if there is no work and no thought following it. Errors in every new program are bound to occur and, unless they are picked up and remedied, the program must suffer. In the case of sex education, a failure can indeed be serious since there is, in many places, so much controversy attached to the subject.

Many people should be involved in the evaluation of the program—students, parents, teachers, counselors, and administrators. In fact, everyone at all involved in the school might well be consulted. The evaluation should be made in terms of the framework of the total educational program of the school and of the needs of the community.

Basic Steps in Evaluation

A. Are the objectives that have been established appropriate and adequate?

    1. Are the objectives specific enough to give direction to the program?

    2. Are they broad enough to meet the needs of all the children?

    3. Do the objectives need revision?

B. Are the objectives being achieved?

    1. What methods or techniques are available to objectively appraise the program?

    2. What are the subjective appraisals of it? What are the opinions of the people involved?

Who Should Do the Evaluation?

Because the sex education program involves a large number of people and because of its importance to the future of each child, we suggest that the principal designate a committee to evaluate the program. This committee should consist of some individuals who are deeply involved in it and some who are not.

It is suggested that the committee consist of parents, teachers, students, and an administrator. If it meets four times a year to discuss developments as they occur, rather than after the fact, far more can be accomplished. If they find a lack of materials, for instance, these may be ordered and obtained before a full semester is over.

It is also the committee's task to judge whether the objectives are being met, whether the program is providing relevant information. It should also synthesize information obtained from the other sources listed below.

Teacher's Analysis of Sex Education Program

(Filled out approximately three times a year)

1. What concepts have you covered during this period? (These may be copied from your syllabus.)
2. What methods or techniques have you used to teach these concepts?
3. Which have you found to have most impact on your children?
4. Which have you found to be the least effective?
5. What objective appraisals have you made in this area—tests, drawings, questionnaires, biographies? What results did you obtain?

6. What is your honest opinion of the program? Do you feel it needs revision? If so, in what areas?
7. Have you the textbooks you need? If not, which would you like to see ordered?
8. Have you the audio-visual materials you would like to use? If not, what would you like to see ordered?
9. What questions or comments have your children made that show understanding of the subject matter or wholesome attitudes?
10. What questions or comments have parents made in regard to the program?

This survey serves two purposes. It furnishes feedback, and it also encourages teachers because it shows that their work will be noted and appreciated.

Pupil Evaluations

This sex education program is, or must be, made as relevant as possible. It must teach the children what they need to know. How can this be evaluated?

In the first and second grades the evaluation must be subjective, with the teacher's comments sufficing. The teacher should look for clues throughout the school year that will indicate the positive attitudes the children are developing.

By the third grade we can ask the children to fill out questionnaires. Anonymity is worthwhile in this particular situation, since the subject is a delicate one.

You might ask the children to answer the following questions:

1. Make a list of five things you learned in sex education that you did not know before you came into this class.
2. In what subjects would you like the teacher to go into more detail?
3. What other subjects (not covered) would you like to know more about?
4. What did you learn that impressed you most?
5. What ideas did you have that you discovered were wrong and which you changed?

This is just a suggested questionnaire. Each teacher should be free to establish his or her own evaluation device.

Evaluation by the Parents

Do not use very long, involved questionnaires for parents since they may be reluctant to deal with such an involved task. Something of the type following is suggested:

1. Have you been aware of the sex education program through comments by your child at home? If so, are you satisfied with it? If not, why not?
2. If your child hasn't said anything, and a great many don't, have you seen any visible attitudes that you can attribute to the sex education program?
3. Have you spoken to your child's sex education teacher or attended any workshops? What is your personal reaction to the program?
4. Are there any improvements you would like to suggest?
5. Do you feel your child is more able to discuss comfortably topics of a sexual nature, or connected with sexuality, at home since the beginning of this course?
6. Have you gone over the material you received and discussed it with your youngster? (Use this question, of course, only if you have distributed material.)

In addition to this questionnaire, parents will be talking with teachers or administrators. Informal comments can be very important in the evaluation of a program. "That Mrs. Smith is doing a wonderful job in her sex education class," Mrs. Jones said to the principal. "My daughter actually came home and said she would like to help with the dishes. She said she didn't realize how much work I had to do at home until her teacher discussed it in family living class."

Evaluation by Administrators

Because sex education is a new program, and because it is such a controversial one, it is advisable for the principal or one of his assistants to know exactly what is going on in the sex education classes. If the school receives complaints, and the principal can handle them in a knowledgeable manner, then the parents or person complaining can be placated far more easily than if it is necessary to do an investigation because the principal doesn't know what's going on.

Supervisory visits serve another purpose, too. They can help to make the situation more comfortable, and less fraught with the tinge of sexiness. Supervisors should know which texts and audio-visual aids are used and exactly how they are being implemented. Particularly during the first year of this program, it is good practice for the supervisor to keep a close eye on it.

Staff Evaluation

Another possible method of evaluating the program is to hold grade level or departmental conferences involving all members of the staff. At these meetings a recorder should be asked to note the comments of the teachers. An open discussion is possible if it is understood that the purpose of the conference is to improve the program and not to penalize any teacher in any way.

Surveying the Progress of the Program

After the questionnaires are gathered and studied, the committee should determine whether or not the objectives of the program are being met. Were they specific enough or too specific? Do they need revision? Could this revision wait until the next semester or should it be done immediately?

Of course, it is expected that the sex education program will improve year after year—we all learn by our own mistakes and utilize our own experience. Hopefully, too, research within the school will continue, with more information being added constantly to the program in the form of added activities and experiences for the children.

It may also be discovered that errors have been made in choice of staff. There are teachers who cannot handle sex education programs. For their sakes, as well as for the children's, they should be given other subject areas to teach. Again, we must remember that teaching sex education is a very personal matter, requiring tact and a great deal of feeling.

Where a teacher must teach it, if he or she needs help, perhaps it will be found in the workshop situation we discussed earlier in this book. The first year is the most difficult for the majority of teachers. They find that as they feel more secure in what they are doing, they are better able to communicate with the children. Sympathy and understanding on the part of the administration are essential. Many fine teachers are lost to sex education and, indeed, to our entire profession because of a lack of these qualities.

Changes in Student Attitudes

The problem with evaluating a sex education program is that so many of the effects it may have are totally immeasurable. How can one measure a change in a child's attitude? How can one tell if a child is influenced by what is going on in his or her classroom? We recall observing one class; the young woman teacher was seated on her desk, her legs folded under her (she was wearing a pants suit), and every single eye in that classroom focused on her. When the supervisor opened the door, an audible groan went up. The very wise supervisor shut the door and left. That day in the lunchroom he asked one of the boys, "Did you learn anything in that class that you didn't know." "I sure did," the boy replied, and walked away before he could be questioned further. This is the type of education we are trying to make sex education—a very personal, relevant thing, to each and every child. The statistical proof will come later, but we can hardly wait for it. For if our program is to be effective, it must reach the children from the primary grades up through high school.

INDEX